Bach Flower Remedies for Children

Bach Flower Remedies for Children

A PARENTS' GUIDE

Barbara Mazzarella

Translated by Tami Calliope

Healing Arts Press
Rochester, Vermont

To my son, Tommaso,
because he is unique, the most wonderful son anyone could ·
ever wish for; and to all mothers everywhere, in hope that
they already know that every child is, in his or her unique-
ness, the most wonderful child in the world.

Healing Arts Press
One Park Street
Rochester, Vermont 05767
www.InnerTraditions.com

*Note to the reader: This book is intended as an informational guide. The remedies, approaches, and
techniques described herein are meant to supplement, and not to be a substitute for, professional medical
care or treatment. They should not be used to treat a serious ailment without prior consultation with a
qualified health care professional.*

Library of Congress Cataloging-in-Publication Data
Mazzarella, Barbara.
[Fiori di bach per 1 bambini. English]
Bach flower remedies for children : a parent's guide / Barbara Mazzarella:
translated by Tami Calliope.
p.   cm.
Includes index.
ISBN 0-89281-649-X (alk. paper)
1. Flowers—Therapeutic use. 2. Children—Diseases—Homeopathic treatment.
3. Homeopathy—Materia medica and therapeutics. I. Title.
RX615.F55M3713 1997
615'.321—dc21   97-302
CIP

Printed and bound in the United States

10 9 8 7 6 5 4

Text design and layout by Kristin Camp
This book was typeset in Goudy with Bernhard Modern as the display typeface

Healing Arts Press is a division of Inner Traditions International

CONTENTS

Acknowledgments

I thank Milla and Francesca for having "forced" me, by their un-wavering faith, to write this book; Paolo and Sergio, who, like the guardian angels they are, have always nourished my "light," most of all in the difficult moments; and my husband Luciano for his patience and support.

INTRODUCTION

To those of you who wish to better acquaint yourselves with the ideas and methodology of Dr. Bach and the Bach flower system, I recommend reading, in addition to this book, at least one of the many good texts available on the subject. Unless you are already familiar with the Bach flower essences, such supplemental reading is indispensable, since this book deals exclusively with their application to the treatment of children. It is my hope, moreover, that what I have written will pique your curiosity and prompt you to look more deeply into this simple yet fascinating process.

It has not been my intention to reiterate what so many others have written about so well. Most books on this subject, however, relegate the treatment of children to a brief comment or two in the appendix, whereas my entire sphere of study has been in this field. I have worked for more than twenty years in the nursery and elementary schools of Milan, and thus my knowledge of the subject is not scholarly but experiential.

To begin with, I would like to give you some background, and it is my duty and my distinct pleasure to acquaint you with the figure of Dr. Edward Bach, who was born in England in 1886. As a child, Bach was extremely sensitive and a great lover of nature, recognizing in every living thing its fundamental soul: soul of butterfly, of brook, of blade of grass. His level of empathy was such that he felt acutely the sufferings of others—so much so, that at the age of six he had already decided to become a doctor, convinced that the alleviation of suffering was his life's work. Before taking his degree in medicine, he worked for a while in his father's factory, where he came to understand the fear that illness generates in people; in those days, not working meant not being paid, and not being paid meant not getting well.

Originally trained as an immunologist, Bach received his degree in 1912. He later became a homeopath and discovered the "nosodes" that are used in homeopathic medicine to this day; still, he remained unfulfilled.

So Bach, who considered injections a barbaric form of treatment, sought a solution in nature. Like Hahnemann, the father of homeopathy, he based his work on the axiom "Cure the person, not the disease." His intuition led him to explore the possibility that, within the perfect pattern of nature, all human beings contained the potential to cure themselves. Certain in his perception that sickness invariably signified a disequilibrium between personality and soul, he recognized in certain flowers the positive energies and potentialities he had been seeking.

Following this revelation, he abandoned a thriving practice and brilliant career, threw out all his precedent research, and left England for Wales. It was there, in his grandparents' cottage, that he began and ended his great life's work.

At this time he was about thirty and had been diagnosed as having an incurable illness; the doctors gave him three months to live. Instead, he died twenty years later, when he felt his work had been completed.

His was not an easy road. Both traditional and alternative practitioners of medicine blocked his way whenever they could; after all, he was obtaining spectacular results by a simple method within reach of everyone. As the medical establishment was so inimical to his research, he severed all ties with it, relinquishing his title and calling himself an herbalist. He continued his work unperturbed, with little help and very few followers, and announced its completion from his bed in the little cottage, where he died in poverty and serenity.

The foundation of Bach's method is the recognition of various human typologies, each containing characteristics that, when harmonious and in balance, allow us to develop our unique qualities, fulfill our evolutionary purposes, and live in wholeness and health, thanks to our connection with our source Self. Once we are able to hear the voice of our soul and follow its guidance, all we do will be in our own best interests.

Negative emotions such as fear, anxiety, loneliness, anger, distrust, pessimism, and disappointment—and whoever harbors one will harbor many, since one negative state creates another—alienate us from our center, leading us to live in disharmony with ourselves and each other. Losing contact with our inner guide, we walk a hard road, refusing to recognize our own divine spark, our part and place in the cosmic whole. This is when dis-ease intervenes to warn us that something is wrong; if we do not heed it, true disease or illness—"beneficent in itself," says Dr. Bach—will intervene to warn us in a much more peremptory manner that we can and must rediscover our balance.

Bach discovered in certain flowers vibrations specifically adapted to reestablish this equilibrium; for every typology and emotion there is a corresponding flower, which he found after years of painstaking research and exploration.

A flower for each of us? Yes, in the sense that each of us "is" a certain flower—in "flower therapese" we say, "She's really Beech," the way homeopaths say, "He's Pulsatilla." So, we are each a flower; but we can also add other flowers to the mix, and this is where things really get interesting.

Let me give you a simple example. I am Vervain: enthusiastic to the point of exaggeration, always hoping to involve others in what I believe (witness this work), energetic and project-oriented, rather loud, and intolerant of injustice. Right now, however, I particularly need the faith and confidence to carry this book to completion, so I add Larch to Vervain; and since I have many other responsibilities to fulfill and am feeling overextended, I'll put some Elm in my little bottle, as well.

If this is not perfectly clear, that may be all the better in that it will stimulate you to experiment and see what works best for you. I don't place much trust in certainties, as a rule. The one exception, which I suggest you plant firmly within your mind (for it is the mind not the intuition that is forever blocking us), is this: It's no big deal if you administer the wrong remedy. It's like trying to open a door with the wrong key; the door doesn't explode, it just stays shut. The worst that can happen is . . . nothing. The desired effect is not obtained, and you try another remedy.

Here is an example: You are administering Elm to a child because the responsibilities of school weigh heavily on her, and she appears tired and overworked, but she doesn't respond. Then you discover that the true cause is repressed anger toward her teacher; you begin to administer Holly, and little by little the knot dissolves.

Have faith in yourselves and your own intuitive instincts. For help with this, take Larch and Cerato; if you're overanxious to see quick results, take Impatiens.

Bach flower remedies are now widely available from herbalists and homeopathic pharmacies. One small bottle of flower essence is sufficient for a very long time and contains a solution of water and brandy, in which are dissolved and diluted the energetic vibrations of the various remedies. There are thirty-eight remedies in all, plus Rescue Remedy, which is a combination of a number of flowers.

Buy a one-ounce vial with a dropper from the drugstore and fill it up to the shoulders of the bottle with natural mineral water. Add about twenty drops of brandy or hard apple cider as a preservative (diluted to this extent these substances couldn't harm a mosquito), particularly important in summer when heat can putrefy the water. The addition of a little alcohol is especially recommended because you absolutely cannot store these remedies in the refrigerator.

Now add two—and only two—drops of each remedy you've chosen. If you're including Rescue Remedy, add four drops of it. Never combine more than seven remedies; in the case of children, three are usually sufficient. Administer four drops on top of or under the tongue (no more, since it accomplishes nothing) three or four times a day. If this is not possible for some reason, you can dilute the remedy mixture in water or fruit juice.

The cost of preparation is minimal, since with only two drops from the mother bottle you will have prepared enough for fifteen days. If you purchase the full set of thirty-nine remedies rather than buying individual bottles, you will save even more. The purchase itself can be a collaborative effort involving parents, teachers, and caretakers, creating a kind of lending library of flowers.

Human beings are not alone in benefiting from Bach flower essences; they may be administered to cats, dogs, goldfish, and other pets, and even to plants and cut flowers.

I suggest that you read my brief descriptions of the flowers and their corresponding typologies several times in order to comprehend and assimilate them fully. This will help you choose the right remedies when the time comes.

If you have the full set, one way to make this choice is to open all four boxes, call in the patient, and tell him to select one or more bottles, just as he likes. He will probably choose exactly the right kind and in exactly the right number. Too simple? One of nature's great strengths is its simplicity, while we tend to complicate things. Give it a try; or if you feel uncomfortable with this method, trust your own intuition and make the choice in a way that aligns with your beliefs.

Don't worry about unwillingness on the part of your patients. I dare anyone to show me a child who balks at taking "four magic drops." Never call them medicine, because they are not. Call them energy drops, love vitamins, asterix potion, or firewater—whatever your imagination can come up with. You can also add them to drinks, as I've mentioned, or sprinkle them on pillows and clothes, in shoes, and even in the corners of the room.

Length of administration is variable. Generally speaking, children respond more quickly than adults because they have fewer mental barriers and are neither blinded by prejudice nor hampered by expectations. Since we are all unique, everyone will have her own time scheme, her own reactions, and her own flowers, which will change as everything changes and transforms. Then they will return because life is cyclical in nature. A determining factor in length of administration is the seriousness of the problem.

As I have said, most available texts on Bach flower therapy give only a cursory nod to the matter of children. However, I find it useful to start stabilizing balance and fostering harmony in human beings at a very early age. If we use flowers to correct negative states and reestablish equilibrium in children, we may well end up with fewer distressed adults.

It is because I believe this that I've been "hatching" this book, in which you will find, along with quasitraditional descriptions of the typologies and remedies, advice and suggestions, games, guided meditations, and stories. Combined with the energies of the flowers themselves, these things can contribute to the fulfillment of an ideal that I have long carried within me. I believe that we were born to be happy, that joy is the birthright of every living child.

It seems to me that all parents, teachers, and caregivers of children would do well to familiarize themselves with the Bach remedies in order to be able to intervene swiftly, without medical involvement, in crises and emergencies responsive to the flowers' effects.

Bear in mind that desire for attention is often the trigger that sets illness into motion. Remember when your mother brought you orange juice in bed? Even as adults we tend to get sick when we're feeling the need to be coddled. Wanting to be cuddled and hugged and held and loved is nothing to be ashamed of; let us make sure that our children get enough of it all, without having to resort to headaches or upset stomachs.

As far as I'm concerned, Dr. Bach's Rescue Cream is a must in any first-aid kit, whether at school or at home. It is good for just about anything: burns, insect bites, bruises, cuts, and rashes, to mention a few. Rescue Cream is homeopathic and oil-free, is not greasy or smelly, and contains Rescue Remedy and Crab Apple.

Don't forget that Bach flower remedies are not medicines. They do not suppress symptoms but instead inundate the recipient with vibrational energies exactly adapted to the person and problem, thus reestablishing balance.

Use of Bach flowers should start before birth, particularly during the last few months of pregnancy. At this time, Rescue Remedy can greatly benefit both the expectant mother and her unborn child by alleviating tension and fear. Various other flowers are also helpful during pregnancy: Scleranthus for nausea; Crab Apple for fear of dirt, bacteria, or blood; Mimulus if the mere idea of a birthing room is frightening; Olive if the pregnancy is particularly exhausting or the expectant mother is overworked; and so on. Apply the same methodology to choice and administration as in any other circumstance.

Just after birth it is advisable for both mother and baby to take Star of Bethlehem because emergence from the womb is the first trauma we all undergo. Rescue Remedy, which contains Star of Bethlehem, can also be given. Walnut is very helpful during pregnancy and childbirth both for its protective qualities and because it is the flower of change and transition.

Although these essences are preserved with alcohol, you needn't worry about the safety of your newborn. The amount of alcohol contained in the final dilution is infinitesimal since the remedy will consist of only four drops of Rescue Remedy or two drops of any other flower, dissolved in one ounce of water, and administered four drops at a time, four times a day.

If the mother is breastfeeding, she need only take the remedies herself for her baby to benefit from them. Alternatively, they can be sprinkled on the nipples before nursing or added to the milk in the bottle.

During weaning, Red Chestnut, which helps to cut the "umbilical cord," is the remedy of choice for mother and child. Walnut is also helpful, since this is another major time of transition. And don't forget to give Holly to your newborn's brothers and sisters, even if they don't appear jealous at all and seem to adore the baby.

On the following pages you will find my descriptions of the various typologies of behavior. It won't be difficult to recognize the child reflected in each flower or the negative mental attitude in need of correction and balance that each flower addresses.

You will also find an affirmation at the end of each chapter.

These are meant not so much for your children as for you. By working with these affirmations, you will nourish yourselves and develop new insights into the ways you speak and interact with the children you care for.

Since significant messages are often communicated most effectively through metaphor, I have written a small story for every flower. Some of these are directed to you—you will know which ones—but most are meant to be read aloud and shared with your children. Read them before bedtime or the afternoon nap. Feel free to make changes, so that the tale more closely fits the listener. But a word of advice: If your son is named Matthew and has dark hair and green eyes, don't call your hero Matthew and give him dark hair and green eyes. The hero/ine should resemble the child, not reflect him or her with precision; this is how metaphor works. If your daughter loves horses, create an elf that loves riding dragonflies. And let the children themselves change or add on to the stories, for their parts of the tale may provide you with the precious keys to understanding.

The time has come to proceed to the description and interpretation of each condition and remedy. I have tried to be as clear as possible and have used layperson's rather than medical or scholarly terms in the hope that what I have written will be of help to parents, teachers, and other caregivers of children. This book is meant to be a practical working manual, within reach of anyone with an interest in the subject.

THE BACH FLOWER REMEDIES

AGRIMONY

I'm always looking for friends.
I pretend to be very happy, but then
I bite my fingernails or eat snack foods
in secret. Maybe I don't feel truly accepted,
so I play the part of the clown.

Agrimony is for those children who are easily consoled, easygoing, and quick to give in, but who then chew their nails or devour too many snacks. They tend to act very cheerful, yet dwell on things in secret.

Agrimony is also effective in cases of "addiction"—to sweets, chocolate, a blanket, or whatever. These children will yield up their toys without a murmur and never, ever quarrel with their friends. If they do, they become highly distressed, since they seek above all friendship and approval from others.

It is necessary to tell Agrimony children that you accept them just as they are, that they are so good and generous it is a pleasure to be around them. In a positive mood they can be truly joyful and lively, so share their joy and laugh along with them; but don't forget that in negative moods they are tormented by an anxious need to please others and by fear of abandonment. Hypersensitive, they are often overstimulated. These children may also scratch themselves continually, gnaw on their nails, or fret with and twirl strands of their hair.

The basic issue to work on is acceptance, so it is important to pay attention to the words you are using. Agrimony children must be loved unconditionally, so that they may learn to love themselves and to understand that they are sufficient just as they are, that they need not adapt or force themselves to act the clown for other people to like them. Always use affirmative statements, even if you must scold them, making sure to emphasize that it is the action, not the child, that is wrong. "Look how messy you are" reinforces a negative self-image, while "This bedroom is really messy" makes the point without denigrating the child. Inconsequential as it may seem, this can actually prevent a buildup of those negative mental frameworks that so many of us drag around with us all our lives.

Remember that Agrimony is a remedy perfectly suited to childhood, since children tend to conceal their private torments. Whatever we may think, they seek in every possible way to be approved and accepted. It may seem to us that there is no problem, but that is only because the trouble is so often hidden.

When nail-biting is brought on by a crisis of anger or by some particular occasion of distress coupled with rebellion, it is good to administer Agrimony with Holly. Any time some kind of addiction is involved, Agrimony should be supplemented by Walnut, which expedites change and, in the words of Dr. Bach, "shatters the chains." Agrimony with Walnut can help them through teething, while Scleranthus steadies them during schedule changes or travel.

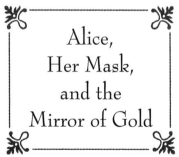

Alice,
Her Mask,
and the
Mirror of Gold

Alice was a lovely little girl like many others, as pleasant and intelligent as any of her friends. But Alice never left the house without first putting on a mask. The truth is that Alice never really felt at ease, but in order to pretend to be happy she glued on this mask with a smiling mouth and laughed like a clown. She laughed so often that even her friends thought her a little bit silly; but since her jokes and funny remarks were amusing, they always invited her over.

Alice couldn't bear to lose out on a single encounter; being with other people was terribly important to her. She had no idea how to be alone, even for a few hours. If she was, it was torture: She bit her nails or ate one snack after another.

Going out without wearing the mask wasn't even an option; by now the mask *was* her personality. And although sometimes the glue on her skin bothered her and gave her a rash, she either wore her smiling mask or she didn't go out at all.

One evening at her friend Elvira's party, as Alice was joking and laughing, she asked herself how Elvira managed to be so unruffled. Although her face was pale and you could see that her curls had come out all wrong, she was calmly enjoying the party, not worrying about a thing.

When the cake was brought out, Elvira's mother took a lot of little packages out of a basket—gifts for the party guests. Alice took her gift and decided to open it later. As soon as she arrived at home, she opened the package; in it was a mirror with a golden frame. She looked at herself and realized that she was still wearing her mask, so she took it off and carefully washed away the glue, applied a little cream to the places that itched, and came back to the mirror.

Now, Alice did not like herself very much, as you will have guessed, and she was a little afraid to look at herself without the mask on. But she thought of Elvira, who had not cared that her curls had all come undone, and she looked into the mirror.

She saw a child with a sad but very sweet face. It occurred to her that maybe no one would want to see her this way, and she began to cry harder and harder, and the tears loosened the knot she always felt in her breast. Finding the courage to look at herself again in the mirror, she heard a voice.

"Just look at yourself, Alice. How beautiful you are! This is the real Alice, not that clown's mask. You are loved just as you are; there's no need to strain yourself so, you have all the rights the other girls have. Tomorrow try to go out with your real face on."

But Alice cried, "Are you mad? If I do, they'll see these pimples from the glue and besides, my eyes are all red from crying. No way! Tomorrow I'm spending all day right here!"

"I promise you that if you go out without your mask, no one will find out about your silly disguise. Besides, a mirror that talks isn't something you can buy at the supermarket, is it? Will you believe me if I tell you that I'm magic—that I've come just for you, to help you understand that the real Alice is better than the masked Alice? If it doesn't work, you can break me into a thousand pieces and go back to the way you were."

So Alice gave it a try.

The first friend that she met in her daring "unmasked" debut said to her, "How glowing you look today! Excuse me for saying this, but usually you just laugh and laugh, and there were times that I thought you were stupid. It's as if I'm seeing you with new eyes today. Do you know that you've changed?"

Alice knew it was not her friend's eyes but she herself who was new, and she realized that the mirror had been right. She went home and polished and thanked it, and the mask and glue ended up in the dustbin.

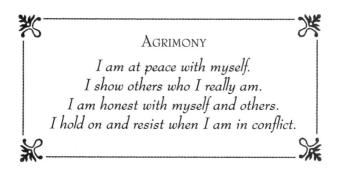

AGRIMONY

I am at peace with myself.
I show others who I really am.
I am honest with myself and others.
I hold on and resist when I am in conflict.

ASPEN

*I have these strange fears—nighttime,
darkness, death. It's hard for me to fall asleep
and sometimes I have terrible nightmares.
I feel anxious and I don't know why.*

Aspen children don't like to be left alone. They are scared of ghosts, robbers, and monsters; they're afraid of the dark and don't want to go to bed at night. TV, of course, encourages and nourishes their insecurities.

Small children, who are still very open, may be in touch with the higher planes, and Aspen helps them to assimilate their experiences without anguish. Take, for example, the imaginary friend. Although a child may actually be seeing something, she is apt to be called crazy or silly if she mentions it to her parents. At times these children are so highly sensitive that they cannot bear to remain in certain places, nor can they stand to be in the presence of some people. It is as if they were breathing in an atmosphere that irritated and disturbed them.

It goes without saying that these fears should not be encouraged; we must take care not to augment them with tales of monsters, evil-doers, or boogeymen. This doesn't mean that we shouldn't read them fairytales, only that we should explain those parts most likely to raise fears in the unconscious and emphasize whenever possible the positive aspects of the story.

It is useless to tell Aspen children that nothing exists outside the material world. Intuitive as they are, they will not believe it, for they feel strongly the invisible dimensions that surround us. Our task, then, is to teach them in the simplest terms how positive their contact with the divine can be.

Here, flower essences can help. Aspen, in combination with Rock Rose, combats nightmares. It can also benefit very sensitive children who claim to see or hear strange things and who are fascinated by fairytales and magic, but later feel uneasy and develop stomachaches. Aspen is, among other things, a remedy helpful to children with mental disturbances caused by abuse (with Star of Bethlehem).

Although it is damaging to encourage their negative fantasies, you can put their desire for magic to use by instigating positive "white magic" rituals that will serve to exorcise many fears. The guardian angel or spirit, the "magic" waters of the full moon, and objects that acquire a spiritual and symbolic value are all powerful tools in their journey toward security.

For instance, if they have problems falling asleep, aside from administering the appropriate flowers (in cases of fear of nightmares try Rock Rose, Mimulus, and Aspen) you can imbue certain objects with protective and talismanic powers. Which one of us does not own an amulet of some kind—a ring, charm, or special stone we love and touch for luck in times of difficulty?

Use your imagination to think up simple gifts bearing beneficent and protective energies. For example, a small magic stone of a certain color or an amethyst crystal for example, may ward away nightmares. Or you might place a little bowl full of multi-colored stones in their bedroom, so that each evening they can choose one to hold in their hands or put beneath the mattress to absorb scary thoughts and transform them into beautiful dreams.

Consistent ritual is a wonderful way to induce peaceful sleep. After they brush their teeth and put on their pajamas but before a bedtime story, have them choose a favorite stone and say a prayer, affirmation, or nursery rhyme; it doesn't matter what it is as long as it's always the same. Depending on your beliefs, you could call on a guardian angel, spirit guide, power animal, or other beneficent being to guard their sleep and protect them from harm.

At Findhorn, a New Age community in the north of Scotland, they use "angel cards" as a way of attracting the energies they need. You can develop your own creativity by getting together with your children and designing some cards especially for them. There are infinite images to choose from; feel free to give rein to your imagination and to that of your children. If an angel is not appropriate, there are elves, fairies, stars, gnomes, and animals to choose from. I have found these special cards to be very helpful. After fishing around in the pile, children can then draw one card to keep in a pocket or backpack or put under a pillow for a touch of magic. Even if you don't believe in them, it is important that the children do (remember Dumbo and the magic feather?).

I use kinds of cards and little notes on which I've written messages or drawn guardian beings, and I have noticed that when I bring them out, everyone starts fishing around for one. They may start out by joking about it, yet end up touched by the infinite divine. After the little ones are tucked into bed, try rummaging around in the bag yourself—you may find a nighttime fairy all your own!

Just think, if we all could be as attentive to our inner child as children are, how beautiful the world would be! Those who believe in magic seldom believe in war; those who "fish" for angels don't want fighter-bomber wings but the wings of angels. If we just listen to our inner child, let her or him play a bit, we too can be as innocent and clear as the children we love.

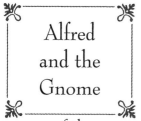

Alfred and the Gnome

Whenever Alfred had to go to bed, he began to shake. No one believed him, but he felt sure that there was something or someone in his bedroom.

Before going to sleep he needed to reassure himself about this. He looked in the corners of the room—but not too hard, because what if in the corner there was . . . ? The door had to be open, but not too much, because what if they came in and . . . ? But if it was closed, how could his mother hear him?

He wanted a glass of water, then a sweet; he was cold, then he was hot; he had a thousand excuses for calling his mama and papa. In reality he just wanted to put off going to sleep.

No one believed him, but he was sure he could hear strange noises. At times he seemed to hear a rustling sound, and then he was afraid there was a snake in his room. Although it was, of course, highly unlikely that a snake would hole up under his bed, that is what he thought. At other times he seemed to hear a kind of squeaking—possibly a mouse? But how could a mouse reach the tenth floor, open a door that was bolted shut, and settle down, baggage and all? Well?

Although Alfred lived in desperate fear, no one believed him; and before he could manage to get to sleep, he had to collapse entirely. Sometimes he woke up from nightmares and screamed until his parents came in to calm him.

Once, however, he fell asleep right away. He had been on a walk in the woods with his papa; they had walked a long time and then played ball. As soon as he hit the bed that night he fell into a deep sleep and had a dream.

In the right-hand corner of his bedroom, right where he kept his skis and ski boots, there lived a little gnome—friendly, cute, and above all, harmless. He had taken up residence in the left boot to stay warm, and he said that his task was to come here from the fairies' world each night and set alight the stars of imagination, creating beautiful dreams in Alfred's bedroom. But before tonight he had never managed to do it. Alfred had always made up so many stories, and such long ones, that the little gnome had always ended up falling asleep first.

It was lucky, he said, that Alfred had taken such a tiring walk today, so that tonight he had been able to fire up this beautiful dream. Otherwise, the fairies would have scolded him again, and he would have lost his job. Yes, it was he who had made all those noises, when he went into the boot or munched on an acorn before going to sleep. But there was no need, he said, to tell mama and papa, because it was a secret between them.

Alfred goes to bed happily now.

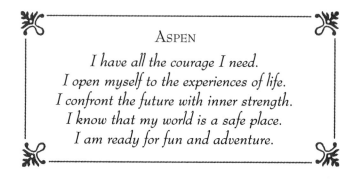

ASPEN

I have all the courage I need.
I open myself to the experiences of life.
I confront the future with inner strength.
I know that my world is a safe place.
I am ready for fun and adventure.

Beech

*The other children say I'm a pain in the neck.
Well, I'm a little critical, but I take things seriously
and I wish that all the others were like me. It's true:
I'm not tolerant. I always see the errors of others,
so they avoid me!*

These faultfinders can always find something to ridicule at home
or at school and are intransigent even with themselves. If a drawing doesn't come out as well as expected, they will fly into a rage;
if they can't find the toy soldiers in the drawer, they will rant
about it for hours. They do *not* like that sweatshirt, neither do
they like Theresa's hair, and they go about airing these grievances
emphatically. In play they try to direct all the games, since they're
the only ones who understand the rules and not to follow the
rules would be to court disaster. The others are so careless!

Beech children can be very quarrelsome; other children may
feel intimidated and avoid them. They can be real bullies, rectify-
ing every situation by imposing their own point of view. They
need to learn that it is all right to have and recognize personal
limits, since this will help them to become more tolerant toward
themselves and toward others.

They must be taught a sense of universality, so that they may
recognize the good in everything and everyone. This is not a difficult task, as children are much more open than we are to concepts
of justice and peace. They are also more directly connected to those
inner voices that nudge us in the right direction for spiritual growth,
both individual and universal. (As we grow, of course, we learn not
to pay attention to our inner voices, with obvious results.)

Urge the Beech child to act without prejudice or bias toward others. Clearly, you must do the same; children are our mirrors and imitate our behaviors, whether they are playing house or scornfully avoiding a not-very-clean or less-than-intelligent child.

Beech in its negative aspect manifests as rigidity. Watch for eventual symptoms of the rheumatic or arthritic type, or more simply, for a stiff neck at an early age. If people are willfully blind to others, choosing to walk down a solitary road, their necks can become as rigid as they are.

This remedy, like Chicory and Vine, can also be helpful in cases of constipation. A controlling child may even feel the need to control physical functions and so hold on.

Beech manifests its positive aspects in those children who can grasp the essentials and make evaluations thoughtfully and objectively. Such children can be of great help to their friends and may be entrusted with tasks in which their clear eyes and critical sense—constructive qualities in this case—will encourage the practice of justice and tolerance in any confrontation.

Because their clarity, reliability, and capacity combine with a deep-seated sense of responsibility, Beech children honor what is expected of them. You can trust that they will always seek out the beautiful and the good. They may function as strong supports for less evolved children since they can give them help and advice in a constructive manner. Because of their positive spirits, they may act as young therapists or teachers.

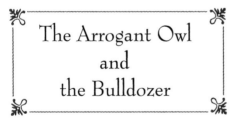

The Arrogant Owl
and
the Bulldozer

In the forest of Forlonia there lived many animals. As is usual in fairytales, they played and conversed with each other. Often they gathered beneath the great oak tree, where Owl read them stories. Owl was the only one who knew how to read; he was highly educated, and he made sure it didn't go unnoticed.

"You should study Latin and stretch your minds," he would say to the Deer leaping about on the rocks. He told Eagle that he flew too high, that he should fly lower; he told Hare not to run so fast, but to study the laws of physics.

"Who could be more foolish than you, Mole?" he would ask. "You're almost blind and you dig holes under the earth. You should study philosophy."

You can imagine how annoying Owl was. When he wasn't reading them fairytales, he had something to say or to criticize every moment. At last he was left alone; no one gathered under the oak, since no one wanted to put up with his constant reprimands.

"Enough is enough," said the animals, and Owl grumbled, "Let them do what they like, the incompetent fools! I have better things to do, I have to translate Tacitus and study logarithms. I'm not ignorant and reckless like they are. We'll see how they turn out!"

Then a very bad day came along. Bulldozer wanted to destroy half the forest to make room to build a mall, and the animals wanted to prevent it. Bulldozer told them it wasn't up to him and said that they would have to make a formal petition on official paper, with reference to article two, paragraph B, of the regional forestry laws.

The animals looked at each other and said, "We need to take this to Owl. Only he knows how to read and write—maybe we should learn."

Owl worked tirelessly on the matter, preparing documents and appeals, making notes in the margins of his papers. But the fatal date drew near; so Hare, who was so swift, went off to deliver the petition, while Eagle searched far and wide from his high lookout, to see if the excavating engineers were on their way.

They were, so Mole began to gnaw at the tires of their automobiles. He and his friends dug so many tunnels that the men in charge of the excavation began to question the wisdom of trying to build a mall there. Meanwhile, Deer climbed onto all the machines and jumped up and down, and Cicadas sang night and day without stopping until the invaders were completely exhausted and went away.

Nowadays there is a school of reading, writing, and various arts under the big oak tree in the woods. Owl has come to understand that everyone has different qualities and capabilities, all of them useful. If Eagle hadn't flown so high, if Hare hadn't run so swiftly, if Mole hadn't frightened the humans with his holes, Owl's knowledge of law would have been almost useless.

All's well that ends well. In just a little while in Forlonia, Owl's arithmetic class will be over, and Mole's lesson in archeological digs will begin. How beautiful the world is when everyone in it is different!

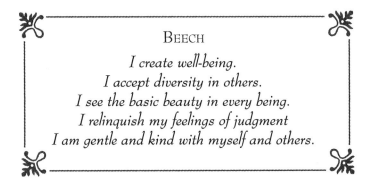

BEECH

I create well-being.
I accept diversity in others.
I see the basic beauty in every being.
I relinquish my feelings of judgment
I am gentle and kind with myself and others.

Centaury

I feel like Cinderella!
I never know how to say no and I always
end up doing whatever the others have decided
I should do. Sometimes I even take on extra tasks.

Submissive and compliant, Centaury children always say yes; they never object or disobey. In school their friends take advantage of them. In large families, they may be elder children, who sacrifice themselves for the others. In any case, this flower acts on the individual's sense of self and works to strengthen the will where there is a lack of self-assertiveness.

Centaury children crave recognition and praise, are extremely sensitive to reprimands, and feel themselves to be somewhat subordinate. In their positive state they are simple and spontaneous, but it is important to help them develop a sense of personal power in its most basic form: "I can." They may never be leaders, but they have to learn not to be doormats. At times they are mentally lazy, finding it more convenient to be little servants than to think for themselves.

It is their self-respect that you need to work with. Praise everything they create and give them "managerial" tasks that will stimulate and stretch their capabilities.

I have to say that in my long years of experience I have never met any Centaury children; perhaps they belong to the past. Education no longer teaches subservience, and ours is an era of freedom of spirit and thought. Understanding comes hard, but we are

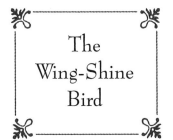

beginning to see that in each of us lie infinite possibilities waiting to unfold.

The Wing-Shine Bird

Everyone else in the flock flew—at high altitudes too—but not the heron, Peppino. His job was to keep the wings of his friends shiny and clean, and he was happy to do it. Just watching the other herons fly filled him with satisfaction. He believed that everyone has his own work: If you have to fly, you fly; if you have to polish and shine, you polish and shine.

It never even entered his mind that his own wings were made for flying. One compliment from the flockmaster and he was happy. He kept his polish and brushes in order and since he made himself the slave of the flock, the other herons nicknamed him Cinderello.

One day a majestic bird with rainbow-colored plumage swooped down in their midst. No one had ever seen such a heron. Who could he be?

Peppino asked him if he would like a good wing-shine or feather-massage, but he answered, "Certainly not! I've come to fly with you."

"With me? No, no, I don't know how to fly, I'm Peppino the wing-shine bird."

"Also known as Cinderello, right?"

Peppino felt sad, but he thought, "I do my duty, I sacrifice myself for everyone else, and now he makes fun of me!"

"Look, I can read your thoughts," said the beautiful bird. "I'm not making fun of you when I invite you to fly with me. It's you who puts yourself down. Whoever told you that just because you tend to the wings of others, you can't use your own?"

"But I've never done it, it's too hard. Just leave it be."

"Peppino, this is your chance. And I have no time to lose; I have to wake up so many others like you! Hurry up now, tidy up your wings as you do so well. Then come over onto that slope with me, and you'll fly like the rest of the herons!"

Peppino felt shy and frightened. This was not something he had ever expected to happen, but to tell the truth . . . he had often dreamed of being able to fly. Now there was nothing to do but decide to say yes, so he puffed up his chest and shouted out, "I want to fly!"

While he was working his way toward the slope he was joined by the flockmaster, Thunder, who said, "Peppino, would you give me a quick once-over?"

Peppino trembled; how could he say no to their leader? Then he felt the kind eyes of Thunder upon him and realized that he, too, wished to see Peppino fly at last. From someplace deep within himself he found the courage to say, "No, sir, now I'm going to fly. Maybe later."

Thunder and the heron of a thousand colors winked at each other, and it was done. Peppino unfurled his wings and launched himself into the air—and so into freedom.

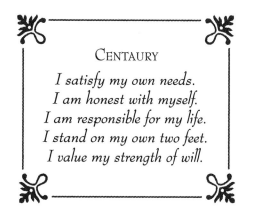

CENTAURY

I satisfy my own needs.
I am honest with myself.
I am responsible for my life.
I stand on my own two feet.
I value my strength of will.

CERATO

I'm always asking advice from the others.
I can't manage to decide for myself because I don't
trust myself. I want to fit in and have the same things
that everyone else has, even if I don't like them.
Sometimes I copy the way my friends dress and talk.

Cerato children are forever asking if what they have done is all right; they have no faith in themselves. At school they crave constant confirmation from the teacher and give the impression, at times, of being a little "slow" to reach their own conclusions. But they are not "slow" at all, only insecure. Because they desire above all to fit in, they will often imitate their companions; rather than take the initiative in schoolwork or play, they will lie low and follow others' leads.

At school they tend to erase what they have written, even when it is correct. Sometimes they know the answer very well but don't dare to raise their hands, since it seems so unlikely that they should be right.

They generally buy the same toys and games that their friends do, or desire those suggested by high-pressure ads, when what they really want is something entirely different. They will ask for the latest video game just to be like "everyone else." In fact, they are not comfortable with diversity, understanding it as negative rather than beautiful and human.

Try to help them see how lovely it is, how wonderful it is to be an individual, and how boring it would be if we were all alike. Work with this concept above all, so that they may begin to perceive how precious their beings and feelings are. With your encouragement, they may learn to trust their inner voice and give freedom to their thoughts.

Cerato children are often starved for information. They want to know, to understand, and ask advice from everyone. This is not always a good thing because it can be a way of delegating choices and decisions to others. Children who are always changing their minds, living in ambivalence and doubt, can make excellent use of Cerato.

In your games and stories, emphasize that all the major human discoveries have come about because someone found the courage to follow his or her intuition. Use examples to help them accept the beauty of individuality, citing their own favorite heroes. Robin Hood, for instance, did what seemed right to him. And if Thomas Edison had listened to the counsel of others, who would have invented the light bulb?

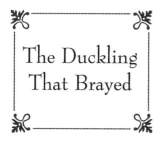

The Duckling That Brayed

Once upon a time there was a farm, and on this farm there lived a lot of animals, of course! Poldo was a duckling, bright and vivacious, but always on the lookout for someone to imitate. When he passed by the barn and saw the cows, he tried to moo; when he heard the sheep, it made him want to bleat.

Now, word went round the farm that Poldo was stupid. Although it's not nice to call someone stupid, that was what they all thought of him. A duck is not a horse; he can swim but not gallop. Yet Poldo insisted, he wanted to learn. He asked advice on how to hold his beak so that he could bray like a donkey. Mama Duck suggested imitating a duckling, but you know how it is, you hardly ever listen to your mother.

One day a gorgeous peacock appeared at the farm. I don't need to tell you that Poldo spent the following week trying to fan his tail—in vain, of course. This peacock was very wise for he had spent many months in a magic and mysterious valley, and he had such marvelous tales to tell that the animals all stayed to listen.

Poldo was always first in line to hear them, and one day the peacock turned to him and asked him point-blank: "Tell me, Poldo, what animal is it that lays eggs, swims in the pond, flies well, has webbed feet, a yellow beak, and multicolored feathers, and says, 'Quack, quack'?"

"A duck?" asked Poldo, who was never sure of himself.

The peacock spoke only one solemn word: "Yes." But Poldo got the message and from that day on he was finally a duckling, one hundred percent.

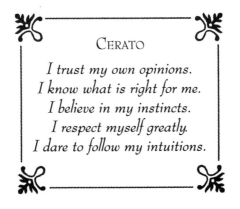

CERATO

I trust my own opinions.
I know what is right for me.
I believe in my instincts.
I respect myself greatly.
I dare to follow my intuitions.

CHERRY PLUM

*I don't tell anyone, but at times I have the most
terrible thoughts; I feel like I'm sitting on a bomb that's
about to explode. I try to control myself, but at times I fly
off the handle and just wish everyone would disappear.
How I frighten myself!*

Cherry Plum children almost certainly suffer or have suffered from
bedwetting. What they manage to control during the day becomes
loosened at night. They may have attacks of rage, obsessive attach-
ments, or phobias. They play the same game over and over; they
wear the same blue overalls every day and resent having them washed.
They want to have everything under control, so they will rummage
around in your purse or drawers with a mixture of suspicion and
curiosity. They pace continually, are twitchy and jumpy, and at times
may actually beat their heads against the wall or furniture.

Cherry Plum can help autistic or psychotic children; it is also
recommended for cases of stammering due to excessive self-con-
trol (there are other remedies helpful for stuttering due to timidity and other causes). To restore the use of speech after trauma,
Cherry Plum is used in tandem with Chestnut Bud. It is also very
beneficial when children cry and scream uncontrollably in a hys-
terical manner or, on the contrary, when they manifest a mania
for order, lining up everything perfectly from pencils to silverware
and folding and smoothing to perfection the cuffs of their shirts.

You must understand that those who require this remedy feel
that they are sitting on explosives. This is why they try to control their every movement—they feel that at the slightest jolt
everything will explode. They may be those apparently "perfect"

children who one day suddenly turn and bite a friend for bumping into them, so hard that they draw blood.

These children neither acknowledge nor express their fears. In essence they are afraid even of themselves and their thoughts, and so they remain silent. The word "relaxation" doesn't exist for them; but it is here that we can help them with activities in which they can let themselves go. We can introduce to them several fine relaxation techniques under the guise of games—massage, sand play, and the manipulation of clay. We should habituate them to listening to sweet and soothing music.

In addition to helping them to relax, engage them in games whenever possible that will help them express aggression in a controlled situation, rather than waiting for a crisis. Let them punch the pillows, wrestle, shout, and yell for an agreed-upon period. Allow them to throw their energy into very fast popular dances where they can stamp their feet and clap their hands. Encourage them to take on small carpentry projects—banging all those nails with a hammer is a wonderful way to work off steam!

In the most serious cases, it's obvious that Cherry Plum must be taken in conjunction with other therapies, whether medical or psychological in nature. I certainly can't claim that the flower itself will heal pyschosis, even if Dr. Bach said, "The illness melts away like snow under sun." There are always constitutional and environmental factors to take into consideration, which may require the help of a psychiatrist or expert in child psychology.

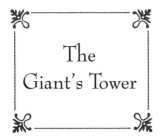

The Giant's Tower

A giant lived in a tower full of furniture and big chests of drawers, which he was wont to stuff with every sort of knick-knack. It wasn't only that he saved everything, even what was useless, he also wrote page after page, describing all of his angers and fears. And then, bang! he closed them away in a drawer; no one else was supposed to see them.

The tower appeared to be very neat, since all the rubbish was hidden in closets and drawers, while everything you could see was in perfect order. Things were arranged according to height, from shortest to tallest. The coffee cups were all turned so that their handles faced left; the jugs were lined up so that their handles faced right. And no one had better challenge the system; the giant had his own way of doing things and would allow no one to change them.

He didn't receive many visitors, anyway, since he was so nervous and quick to anger, always brooding and suspicious of everyone. Though big and strong, he was at heart a sad little man, with all those fears shut away in drawers so full they threatened to burst.

He bought more wardrobes and bureaus 'till the tower swayed and buckled under the weight of them all. But he was oblivious to the danger, more afraid of letting go than of anything else. At times he was tempted to throw out or burn it all. It wasn't easy to keep that enormous amount of stuff in order and under control, yet he couldn't bring himself to do a thing about it.

One day, however, a thunderstorm settled the matter. While the giant was running around in his garden, where he had hung out an enormous load of laundry (socks arranged by color, shirts by size and style), a bolt of lightning struck the tower. Since it was already shaky and overloaded with junk, it came tumbling down and collapsed into a pile of rubble.

The giant wept, shouted, screamed, and kicked at the stones. "Poor me," he cried, "I'm left with nothing, nothing! All my memories, all my papers, all my precious odds and ends!" And as he went on yelling and crying, all the fears that he had kept shut away in those drawers began to come out and make themselves known.

After a long time, when he had gotten them all off his chest, he began to feel as though he had just been set free. He could start over, he could build himself a smaller and more cheerful tower, less burdened by furniture—maybe he could even move. He felt suddenly lighter and said to himself, "Why not?"

He gathered up his shirts and socks and found a backpack and his sack of silver coins among the rubble. Then he set off whis-tling for a new destination, without even looking behind him. The tower had kept him in prison for so long! Now it was just a heap of jumbled-up stones, and he was a brand-new man.

CHERRY PLUM

I remain strong under great stress.
I am calm and courageous.
I choose to be balanced and stable on every occasion.
I am as strong as a rock.
I do what is right.

CHESTNUT BUD

*How tiring school is. I make the same mistakes
over and over. I feel like I study but nothing sticks. I
don't understand things. I must be slow. And now that
I think about it, it's not just in school: I always trip over
the same old rock; I always buy clothes
that I never put on.*

This is a very useful flower for young students who have difficulty understanding their lessons or who frequently repeat the same errors. While the Cerato child will erase an answer even if it is correct, children in need of Chestnut Bud have no idea that they have made a mistake. They are often distracted; they trip over the same thing time after time; they love to repeat the same phrases, the same old joke—and are often avoided or made fun of by their companions, who are bored by their repetitive behavior.

They never manage to work through their errors; they just go ahead and repeat them. They have always forgotten their notebook and left it at home; they can't seem to concentrate and show very little interest in school. Their spatial/temporal reality is actually different than other people's, usually slower, so that they are unable to coordinate their inner and outer worlds. Their answers to questions often seem inadequate, even "stupid," and their teachers are forever warning them: "Think before you speak!"

Chestnut Bud benefits autistic and retarded children as well as those affected by Down syndrome, since it aids in comprehension. Administration of this flower is also beneficial in cases of recurrent or cyclic illnesses because the principle is the same: We haven't understood the "lesson," which will continue to present itself until we do.

Dr. Bach included Chestnut Bud in his remedy for taking exams because of its capacity to restore the powers of concentration and comprehension. It is also indicated for anyone who resists growing and learning: for all the Pinocchio's and Peter Pan's, regardless of age.

We must instill in these children a love of learning and a joy in all that is new, through "heuristic" games of discovery. We must provide them with opportunities to evaluate and discover and encourage them to become curious; there are infinite ways to do this.

Surprises are wonderful, since they need to learn to enjoy being amazed; so are puzzles and riddles, games in which it's up to them to find the error. Choose-your-own-adventure books, with their array of options and ways to solve mysteries, are great and are available in any good children's bookstore.

Again, don't confuse this way of being with that of the Cerato child, who erases even what is right. Remember that the Chestnut Bud child doesn't know she has made a mistake, and instead of a hunger for information, manifests repetitive behavior.

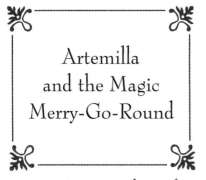

Artemilla and the Magic Merry-Go-Round

Artemilla was a fairy, very small and luminescent, with golden wings and a rather mouselike face. Like all the other fairies, she went to school to learn magic, but without much result. Once she had learned a spell, rather than going on to something new, she just made the same magic over and over for months. Naturally, she wasn't very popular; no one was interested in her enchantments since they were always the same. The truth is, she wasn't very attentive during class, didn't seem to realize it when she made a mistake, and was forever changing the same old toad into a prince—and who can't do that?

The other fairies were amazing; every day they came up with new and wonderful spells and their wings became ever more brilliant. Their followers clapped and cheered them on. Meanwhile, Artemilla was stuck where she was and didn't even seem to know it. She thought she was studying and she went to class, but every day on her way to school she tripped over the same jasmine bush, so that she always had a band-aid on her elbow.

Now, the fairies' teacher felt that the time had come to do something special for Artemilla. The way things were going, she would never earn her regulation wand, and the other fairies would continue to avoid her. Drawing on her store of magic arts, she took Artemilla and set her down on a clock's gear like a merry-go-round. She started it spinning and as it whirled round, she chanted this spell:

> The clock's hands turn and spin and sing,
> And golden are her little wings;
> Swift as an arrow fly, and straight,
> For she is slow and she is late
> To learn the lesson cannot wait;
> Sprinkle her with common sense,
> Give her fresh magic to dispense;
> Banish all that's old and trite
> That what is new may come to light;
> Whirl, little wheel, spin fast
> So that the spell you weave may last.

When the strange merry-go-round came to a halt, Artemilla was dizzy and dazed, and there was a tingling in her head and wings. At once she felt the desire to turn an elephant into a violet. It turned into a tulip instead, but she wasn't discouraged; she finally understood that you can learn from your mistakes, and on the third try she was successful. How the other fairies cheered and clapped!

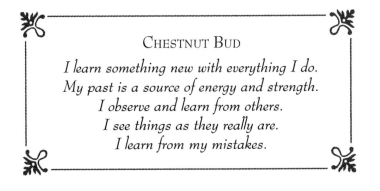

CHESTNUT BUD

I learn something new with everything I do.
My past is a source of energy and strength.
I observe and learn from others.
I see things as they really are.
I learn from my mistakes.

CHICORY

I like little children so much—I like to mother them.
Even when I was little I was always the teacher. I have so
much to give! Naturally, I expect some gratitude in return.
And my friend (if she is my friend) makes me feel very
jealous when she does certain things; she should
pay attention to me, right?

"It's mine!" Possessive and extortionist, Chicory children want everything and everyone to revolve around them. They lend nothing, let go of nothing; on the contrary, they are always demanding treats, gifts, and attention. They will even fall ill to ensure that others will be at their beck and call. These young tyrants use sickness to garner sympathy and keep everyone under their thumb. They cry often, are prone to constipation, and tend to dramatize every situation.

Jealous of their possessions and affections, these children have unfortunately already absorbed, through no fault of their own, the concept of "I'll give it to you on one condition." For example, they may kiss their grandmother (often a Chicory personality too) but only in exchange for three cookies or a new toy car.

Chicory can manifest as an unhealthy attachment on an oedipal level between mother and son. In such cases it is helpful to combine this remedy with Red Chestnut. Chicory should be used in combination with Holly in cases of jealousy, particularly when a newborn sibling is taking up mother's attention.

Girls in need of this remedy are those sweet "little women" who take such good care of the little ones as long as they do everything they want. They suffocate younger children with kisses, cuddle and pet and make much of them, but all this affection comes at a very high price. In fact, if one of their little darlings tries to move out of their sphere of action, these tender "mothers" turn savage and vindictive. They are simply following the model they know, preparing themselves to become overbearing and suffocating parents.

Chicory children are easily recognizable even in play because they always choose the lead roles: teacher, nurse, Mother Courage. In their relationships with others, all sorts of difficulties arise, springing from possessiveness and jealousy and the expectation of what they deserve in return. They fall into a tragic mode if their best friend eats lunch with someone else and are wildly jealous if a schoolmate is praised by the teacher for some group effort in which our "hero" gave all and the other child, nothing—for that is how they perceive it.

All in all, a lot of work needs to be done to help these children. To begin with, their parents need to examine and make changes in their own behavior, since they are perpetuating an erroneous concept of love. Love for its own sake, love for the pleasure of loving, is what Chicory children must learn. Giving them an animal to care for—not to enslave, but to cherish—is a wonderful way to do this.

What they need to develop is a sense of universal love, embracing plants, flowers, birds, stones, and human beings. Why not involve them in some kind of project of help and exchange with children who are less fortunate than they are? You may find them happy to give energy and even a little of their allowance to the cause without expecting anything in return.

Don't encourage them in conditional exchanges: "If you get a good grade I'll buy you those sneakers," for example. If you plan to buy them the shoes, buy them and be done with it; otherwise the relationship becomes a ping-pong game of sweet extortions and more or less veiled blackmail.

In its positive manifestation, Chicory is linked to the principle of unconditional love, on which we must all reflect and to which we must all aspire. Let us remember that this divine love can only flow from us once we have learned to love and accept ourselves to the very core. How else can we love others without limit? When we learn to live our lives from that place, without expectations, all will come to us in its time, unfolding in its perfection.

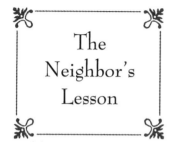

The Neighbor's Lesson

Catherine's house was like a mirror: Her floors and furniture shone brilliantly, her curtains were snow-white, and all her little knick-knacks were of the most expensive kind. She did all the housework herself and kept everything in perfect order. Her neighbor was another story. It's not that she was slovenly, but she tended to get through her household chores in a hurry. In her free time she read books and took lessons in ballroom dancing.

Catherine disapproved and frequently offered unsolicited advice; she was sure she was the only one who knew how to fold napkins and iron shirts correctly. She still ironed all her sons' shirts, although they were grown men and married; she claimed that her daughters-in-law ironed badly as a consequence of having careers. But even as she did it, she complained, saying it hurt her legs to stand so long.

Her neighbor said, "Well, then, don't iron! Come take dancing lessons with me—they're fun and they strengthen the legs."

"As if I had time to waste like that," grumbled Catherine, "I'm a good mother and sacrifice myself for my children."

"Yes, but then if you complain and feel badly. . . Look," said her neighbor, "I have children, too, whom I love very much, but I raised them to be able to take care of themselves. Maurice, who's off studying in London, cooks, cleans, and does his own laundry. Eliza works as an airline flight attendant, so I don't get to see her too often, but I know she's happy and doing well and that's enough for me."

Catherine was scandalized: one child always up and down in airplanes and the other one living alone and so far away! "Oh, no, that wouldn't do for me," she said. "I convinced my children to stay right here in the neighborhood. They come to eat dinner with me every Sunday—or else! I spend hours preparing chicken with stuffing and apple pies."

"But listen," interrupted her neighbor, "don't you think it might be better if once in a while they could just go about their own business? I don't mean to meddle, but every Sunday you all look so unhappy! And afterward you always have some new tale of trouble to tell. Let them live their own lives! You might see them less often, but they'd be more cheerful if they came when they chose to come."

"That's enough, you good-for-nothing woman. Mind your own business," shouted Catherine, deeply offended. "You can talk, you egotist, you're so busy dancing and reading trash you don't bother to find out how your own children are doing! You're a degenerate mother, don't speak to me again!"

"I didn't mean to offend you, only to help you. But if you keep on clucking at your children as if they were chicks. . . ."

"I told you to keep your mouth shut!" shouted Catherine, and she stomped off, slamming the door behind her.

A few hours later her neighbor's telephone rang. Catherine, who never was one to mind her own business, pressed her ear to the wall and heard her neighbor say, in a loving voice: "Of course, Eliza, you and your friend can come for Easter. . . . No, don't worry, I'll do it. . . . Yes, I made you that pink sweater you liked so much. . . . No, I am not tired. I'm even taking dancing lessons. . . . Oh, you two make me so happy—you're such wonderful kids. Maurice is coming on Saturday. . . . Yes, didn't I tell you? He's arriving with his British fiancée, and just as a surprise I've been studying a few British phrases. . . . Well, who knows, but it comes from the heart. You know, speaking of heart, today I tried to help Catherine, who lives next door. I was trying to make her understand you can't own the people you love. I'm afraid I just made her angry, poor thing! She's already so full of problems and sorrow, I was hoping I could be a friend, but hey, she probably won't even talk to me now. Ciao, my sweet, I'm going to hang up now or you'll spend a fortune."

Catherine felt so strange she was almost frightened. So that's how it was; she had understood nothing. Her neighbor wasn't the self-centered person she'd taken her for—not at all. She was loving and loved by her children. Now what should she do?

Standing there with her ear to the wall she was changed; the message got through. She walked over and knocked on her neighbor's front door. "Excuse me," she said, "if I was a little brusque. When's your next dance lesson? You know, if it's really good for the circulation. . . . I was thinking that my daughters-in-law might be able to take those shirts to the drycleaner's or iron them on Sundays if they stayed home instead of coming here. I was even thinking, if you wanted to, we could go to the movies together."

The two women held out their arms and moved toward each other and hugged each other hard. And so began a great and lasting friendship; such is the power of unconditional love.

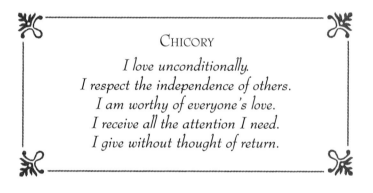

CHICORY

I love unconditionally.
I respect the independence of others.
I am worthy of everyone's love.
I receive all the attention I need.
I give without thought of return.

CLEMATIS

*"Where in the world are you?" people ask me.
And it's true that I'm off in the clouds a lot. I get
distracted, I lose things, forget things. I like to dream, to
draw and paint, to fantasize—but then I find out I'm
late for school, and not only that, I've brought
the wrong books!*

Always distracted, Clematis children have their heads in the clouds. Without meaning to, they disrupt the class by being so vividly elsewhere. When the teacher calls on them, they may not answer; they're busy chasing their dreams or watching a fly circle round. They are not the lazybones they appear to be. It's just that their inner worlds, so rich and fantastic, are much more fun than the classroom!

They draw beautifully and with great imagination, but their senses of sight and hearing are not always what they should be due to their self-imposed isolation. They have a deep fascination with the future and spend more time with space robots and time machines than in the here and now. They lose things, even things it would seem impossible to lose. They get so distracted that they fall out of their chairs; they are sleepyheads.

Clematis is an important component of Rescue Remedy and the remedy for exams. It is the flower that grounds us, brings us back to the earth and helps us plant our feet there.

Clematis children can be rather pale and suffer from cold hands and feet. Their lack of interest in the present can lead to a lack of appetite as well and when they fall ill, recovery can be a long and arduous affair.

They benefit from all activities that bring them into contact with the earth: dancing, gardening, sack races, sculpting in clay, whatever keeps them from flying away into their fantasy worlds. They need a diet rich in high-energy foods, and a piece of chocolate now and then is not only a treat, but a good idea.

Don't tear down their castles in the air. Rather, encourage them to integrate their imaginations with reality so that fantasy may help them to transcend insecurities and fears. Stimulate them in an artistic sense, giving them opportunities to express their inner lives through painting, drawing, and other forms of art.

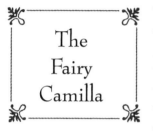

The Fairy Camilla

To be a fairy is a wonderful thing, and Camilla was glad to be able to fly high above the clouds—always higher and farther. Way, way below her spun the tiny world, while she flew through a sky filled with rainbows. Her enchanted hands designed drawings in gold, luminous, heavenly paintings in which colors and stars melded together in fantastic whorls and swirls.

But Camilla often forgot even to eat. Sometimes she flew so hard and so long that later she had to sleep for hours and hours. At times she skipped her magic lessons, and when someone asked her a question, her answer was absentminded or made no sense at all. "Where in the world are you?" people would ask, but she was way out there, not in the world. Everyday things didn't interest her; she preferred to drift in the blue. She was a dreamer, an artist, and only in infinite space did she feel herself.

One day, however, Camilla fell ill. Luckily it was nothing serious, just a bad case of tonsillitus, and the fairy herbalist prepared her a special herb tea. But not only did she forget to drink it, she flew away without it! Of course, this made her condition worse and kept her tonsils from healing, but she seemed not to care whether she healed or not.

So the fairy herbalist decided to sit by her bedside, to keep her from flying away and to help her get better, but after a while she realized that Camilla could fly even inside her mind. She truly didn't want to stay on this earth, not for one moment.

"Would you mind telling me why you're always up there?" asked the herbalist. "You're not a bird, you know. So, you can fly, but you still have to live and learn on this earth. What's going on?"

"I feel good up there. When I'm way up high, I see so many beautiful things, fabulous things, all kinds of colors."

"But they're down here, too. Look outside your window, do you see the flowers? Would you call them beautiful, colorful even? Touch the grass, touch the earth, think how miraculous it is that a tiny seed can do so much! In the sky there are stars and clouds, it's true, but how much else? Have you tried working in the garden?"

The herbalist did all she could to interest Camilla in everyday things. They planted anemones and carrots; they made cakes shaped like stars and sweet breads shaped like hearts. She showed her the magic a needle and thread can make and taught her that fabulous art can be made out of anything, from flower petals to buttons. Why did she do all this? Because she knew that Camilla was in danger of flying away and never coming back at all. Her sojourns in the sky must be briefer; her feet must touch the ground, at least once in a while.

To make quite sure this happened, the fairy gave Camilla a pair of golden shoes, very lovely but also very heavy, so that after her fantastic flights she would come back to earth and rest. You know how it is . . . the end justifies the means.

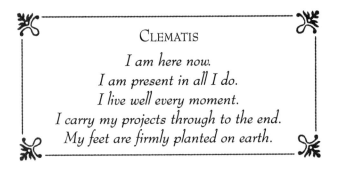

CLEMATIS

I am here now.
I am present in all I do.
I live well every moment.
I carry my projects through to the end.
My feet are firmly planted on earth.

CRAB APPLE

*I'm always washing myself. I have a horror of germs,
bacteria, and bad smells, and I never use the bathroom at
school! I like everything neat and orderly, I like my clothes
to be superclean, and as for my body—well, it's kind of
embarassing. I dress in things like overalls that don't
show my shape, but what about when I become a young
adult? Won't it be disgusting?*

Shower, shampoo, brush, and comb—Crab Apple children are
fastidious about their own bodies. They make sure that their nails
are clean, that their sweatshirts don't smell bad. Clean to com-
pulsive excess, they change socks twice a day and cover themselves in powder and cologne. They will never use an unfamiliar
bathroom. Their hands are always spotless because they never
touch the earth unless they have to, and even then they do so
very cautiously, taking great care not to dirty themselves. Silverware and glasses are scrutinized minutely; they require separate
forks for separate foods or polish the used one with their napkin.

This remedy is called for in cases of rashes and other inflammations of the skin as well as for colds and catarrh. In the Bach system it is considered the great purifier. Crab Apple is indicated in
puberty for problems caused by hormonal changes and for adoles-
cent acne. Because of its cleansing action, it is also useful for indigestion (sometimes stomachaches have to do with "letting go") as
well as for allergies, bronchitis, or whatever is in need of cleaning
out.

Children in need of Crab Apple often feel ill at ease, uncomfortable with themselves, not up to par. Unfortunately, our ste-
reotypical perceptions of beauty and attractiveness make it difficult

to live with any little physical flaw: A mole, a pimple, a too-broad nose, or a bit of a belly can be blown out of proportion. They may also suffer shame at having "bad" or "dirty" thoughts from a natural sexual curiosity about the bodies of others. Crab Apple children may feel a sense of shame about their bodies or may have been victims of sexual molestation.

Crab Apple is found in Rescue Cream for external use. The flower essence can also be used in baths or compresses. Two or three tablespoons of water mixed with two drops of Crab Apple make a good purifying lotion. After a regimen of medicinal drugs, it can act as a detoxicant.

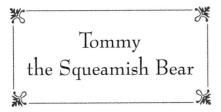

Tommy the Squeamish Bear

It's not easy for a bear to live in the woods and try to keep his paws clean. But for some reason Tommy had a terror of germs. When his fellow bears found a beehive and stuck their paws in it to lick the honey, he made a face of disgust and ran to the brook to wash. The others scooped up big, beautiful fish in their paws; Tommy used a line and hook, and afterward cleaned the fish, removed its spine, and washed it several times before eating it.

His den was extremely clean because he was at war with dust and dirt. He passed his days between huge bouts of den-cleaning and very, very long baths.

Of course, the other bears teased him. It's hardly bearlike to coat your fur with deodorant every few hours. And who doesn't get a little mud on them, living in the forest? And then there was his fear of germs and sickness! Who ever saw a bear who ran to get a blood test or have his appendix taken out, just because he ate a rotten apple?

The time for hibernation was drawing near. All the bears ate until they were practically bursting to fatten themselves up for the long sleep. Tommy, on the other hand, busied himself cleaning his den to perfection and sealing up the windows and every little crack so that germs couldn't get in. He didn't gorge like the others; being chubby made him self-conscious.

In the last days of fall, just before hibernation, the bears stuffed themselves on a certain bitter-tasting weed. "That's disgusting!" said Tommy, and went indignantly into his den, where he brushed his teeth and went to sleep; everything was in order.

After a few days of deep sleep, however, Tommy woke up with atrocious pains in his belly. He didn't know what was happening to him; it hurt so badly! In his fright, he ran to the oldest of the bears and shouted, "Wake up, Bartholomew, I'm sick, I feel bad!"

"Who's disturbing my hibernation? Since when do you wake up a bear who's asleep?" Bartholomew grumbled. "Oh, it's you, Tommy. What's up? Did you finish cleaning your house? Or did you come to tell me you found a fungus in the dust?"

"No, I feel bad, I feel very bad, I have terrible pains in my stomach."

"Yes, no doubt, and if you weren't so squeamish, you'd know you had worms, too."

"No, no, don't tell me that! It's not possible, I hardly eat, I couldn't have worms!"

But the old bear said, "You'd better face the facts, as disgusted as you feel. Listen, three days before hibernation, didn't you eat the bitter weeds to clean yourself out like the rest of us?"

"No, those filthy weeds revolted me."

"All right, my dear bear—if you are a bear—but you should know that since time began we have always cleaned out our bellies with that bitter herb before sleeping. Otherwise we'd have worms and get sick. You are so sterile from head to foot that if an ant left a mark on your floor you'd probably fall ill."

"Am I dying?" asked Tommy in terror.

"No, no, drink this decoction of bitter herbs and in a few hours you'll be fine. Here now, drink it all in one gulp."

Tommy stared at the cup, which didn't look completely clean, and hesitated. But when he looked up, he saw that Bartholomew had raised a huge paw. He knew he was about to be swatted right where he needed it most, so he drank the potion down in one swallow and headed back to his den. This time he went to sleep and didn't wake up until spring.

> ### Crab Apple
>
> *I free myself from every addiction.*
> *I deserve perfect health.*
> *I treat myself with interest and tenderness.*
> *I encourage my body to heal.*
> *I love myself.*

ELM

*I don't know why, but I just can't seem to make
it anymore. Dance class on Thursday, swimming on
Monday and Saturday, and all my homework, too! And I
wanted to direct the theater group. . . . Now exams are
coming up—what will I do? Help!*

When schoolwork, swimming, dance, and language lessons—all
the things you encourage them to do—are obviously just too much
for them to keep up with, relent a little (try taking Pine) and give
them Elm, a support in unsteady or fainthearted moments. During times of intense activity and responsibility—if they must take
exams, write an essay, give a recital, or compete scholastically, for
instance—administer Elm. Children who say, "I'm tired, I can't
handle all this week's homework, it's too much!" need Elm and
possibly a less demanding teacher.

This remedy can help very disturbed children to bear the burden of psychotic material bombarding the ego. Elm is also useful
for so-called growing pains, when the forming skeleton is under
stress.

You can help children under stress by guiding them through
revitalizing relaxation techniques based on breathwork and creative visualization. Don't think they can't do it; it's easier for children than for us. Use scenes from nature, and let the children
draw upon their own inventiveness in finding a vehicle for renewal. It could be a tree, for instance, or a dolphin; the form is
not what matters. The important thing is to train children to journey within themselves, to connect with the source of their own
beings and set into motion the healing energy that they find there.

Creative visualization can also be used in nursery school during rest period, transforming what is often perceived as an enforced, even punitive naptime into a joyous occasion of imaginative flight. (See pages 141–149 for examples of guided meditation.)

Again, the administration of Elm is significantly beneficial during adolescence. It is often arduous for teenagers to keep up with all that is expected of them in the way of schoolwork and chores while they are also experiencing swift physical growth and hormonal changes (add Walnut). Everything is urging them to grow up and become adults, yet they still want to be children; the conflict can weigh on them and wear them down.

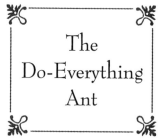

The Do-Everything Ant

There was once a very capable ant, who could carry enormous loads of crumbs and knew how to organize everything so well that the other ants entrusted her with every new job that came along.

"A tunnel needs to be dug for the storage of these cookie crumbs," they would say. "Let's have the do-everything ant dig it out, so we'll know it's done well. She can tally up the grains of rice while she's at it—that way we'll know they've been counted correctly. She's a perfectionist, that one."

So the poor little ant found herself overloaded with work. She didn't receive any help whatsoever, and since she was so responsible, she wore herself out to the breaking point.

"Still, I'm capable of doing it and so I must do it," she would say to herself. "If I don't, who will?"

But finally one day, after carrying and digging and counting and registering—and much, much more—the do-everything ant heard a voice inside herself yelling, "I can't do anymore, it's all too much!" Her legs refused to move and she felt like a mountain was about to fall on her and squash her, but what could she do? How could she not do the work entrusted to her?

Exhausted, she let that inner voice out, and all through the anthill they heard: "Enough, it's too much! I can't do it all myself and I don't want to do it all myself! You have to help me! I don't care if I'm good at it, I'm just tired to death! Do your part, I can't take this anymore!"

For a moment the ants were shocked and amazed, but then they realized that they had gone too far. Of course, they had thought the do-everything ant was happy to take on all these tasks; that's how it had seemed. At any rate, they began to divide up the work once more, as is done in every self-respecting anthill. And with everyone doing his or her bit, no one was overwhelmed.

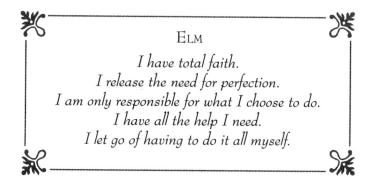

ELM

I have total faith.
I release the need for perfection.
I am only responsible for what I choose to do.
I have all the help I need.
I let go of having to do it all myself.

GENTIAN

*I feel sad and discouraged. Things always turn
out badly for me, and then I'm so disillusioned! My kitten
is sick, and my grades at school are the worst—
there's no way for me to be happy.
And I can't do anything about it.*

The smallest things can discourage children in need of this remedy. Even the broken arm of a doll or teddy bear can cause them moments of enormous difficulty and discouragement.

Gentian is called for when nothing is going well at school and there is a sense of defeat, and in all times of mourning, to help in recovery from grief. In cases of mourning, always extend compassion and understanding to the Gentian child. Even the little goldfish that dies is a grave loss, because these children are more sensitive and attuned than we are. They are, at this point, utterly devoid of cynicism.

Gentian is helpful during periods of convalescence because it aids in overcoming disappointment and encourages recovery and new beginnings. It is also present in the compound for exams, along with Clematis, Chestnut Bud, Larch, and Elm.

Gentian children are sad and often sick. Bear in mind that illness is frequently a form of escape for them, a way of not having to face reality or certain situations. They may even like being sick so they can say, "I won't ever be happy." They may suffer from allergies, actually attracting pollen by virtue of their pessimistic thinking: "I knew I'd feel awful, that's just the way it is!"

They are generally closed and withdrawn and are careful not to get interested or involved in things, though such involvement would go far toward solving the problem. Sedentary by nature, they are not fond of activities that require an expenditure of energy.

More than anything else, Gentian children need to develop their powers of positive thought. You can help them to gain faith by giving a little nudge to the wheel of fortune. If, for example, you had someone strongly visualize a certain outcome and then it came about . . .

Finally, help them with music. Joy without music and song is like a gray and beige rainbow.

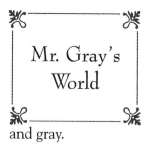

Mr. Gray's World

Mr. Gray was never happy. His mouth seemed stuck in a frown, and nothing that happened pleased him. If the sun was out, he said, "What a nuisance the sun is!" but if it rained, he said, "Oh, no, it's raining again!" Everything he touched became sad and gray.

Not that everything always went smoothly. Occasionally, he had practical reasons for being discouraged. But he actually looked for problems; he knew ahead of time just what to do to ruin a beautiful day. Was that a rainbow coming his way? Oops! He touched it, so that he could say, "How sad! It's all gray!" He didn't understand that it was he himself who was gray.

His neighbor, Peter, was just the opposite. When the sun was out he was glad to turn somersaults in the meadow, when it rained he amused himself by splashing around in the puddles, and if a rainbow came his way, he slid right into it, so as to be covered in colors. He didn't see life in shades of gray.

Mr. Gray didn't find any reason to be happy, and he didn't try to find one either, preferring to sit around and sigh. Peter managed to color everything with gaiety and cheer and enjoy every moment.

You who are listening know that this story has no beginning or end. It's a big sign with a message: Take all the grays out of your life. The world is full of colors: Use them!

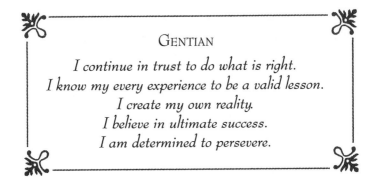

GENTIAN

I continue in trust to do what is right.
I know my every experience to be a valid lesson.
I create my own reality.
I believe in ultimate success.
I am determined to persevere.

GORSE

I have no hope! Don't you see what's happened to me? I can only live in despair, there's nothing else left for me—it's the end.

In a perfect world, Gorse would never have to be given to any child, but unfortunately, even children can be chronic invalids or incurably ill. Sad as it is to think of, there are children on their deathbeds who are in need of help. In such cases, Gorse can relieve the sense of hopelessness.

Pale, sallow, blemished skin, hollow eyes, and drooping lids are all characteristics that may be seen in children existing in situations of great poverty and difficulty. They are bearing heavy burdens and lack the life force typical of their age; they seem like little old people.

Gorse is indicated in cases of severe failure from which there seems no hope of recovery and during great misfortune, when hope is lost. It is helpful to handicapped children, who have a difficult and arduous karma to live out.

Such children need plenty of sun and joy in their lives, along with a nutritious diet rich in energy foods. They need to laugh and to feel loved, to understand that a joyous life is possible in any situation. You can help by exposing them to gay, happy music and upbeat movies and theater. Surround and clothe them in cheerful colors. Fill their hands and pockets with confetti on occasion, to turn an ordinary day into a party. Help them to live in courage rather than in self-pity; they need to feel that they can stand alone. All the capacity, all the potential is in them—help them to blossom.

Never underestimate the resources available to children in need of this remedy. We must live in the faith that some things are beyond comprehension and transcend the scope of reason and that every life on this earth, as Dr. Bach said, is simply a page in the book of our lessons. Surely many souls who labor under weighty and difficult incarnations are fulfilling a divine plan, whose dimensions outstrip our capacity to perceive them.

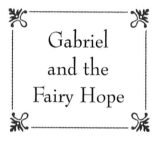

Gabriel and the Fairy Hope

Gabriel was an elf, and he was very sick. This doesn't usually happen to the inhabitants of the fairy world, but as we all know, you only have to imagine something and it can occur.

Now, Gabriel had fallen out of a tree, and after being in a cast for three months, he got it in his head that he would never walk again, and so it was. Of course, after such a long time of not moving, it wasn't easy to start up again. But he didn't even try; he felt that his life was over. The chief of the elves brought him potions and ointments, and Gabriel used them, but they had no effect, since he no longer believed he could heal. He didn't go to parties anymore, and he ate almost nothing.

"Look, Gabriel, it's not as if you sing with your legs! Come to the full-moon festival and play on your flute. You used to make such beautiful music," invited the elves. But even when he let himself be dragged to a party, he wouldn't play his flute, or sing, or laugh. It seemed that he was just waiting to die, and that's exactly what he was doing.

One evening during the festival of the crickets, a friend asked him how he came to be in such a sad condition, and why he didn't try to walk again or at least to sing and make music. Gabriel answered in a feeble voice, "I have no hope. . . . There is no hope at all."

It was as if he had just pronounced a magic spell! An immense light appeared before him, and he heard a tinkling of little bells and laughter. He opened his eyes wide and saw a most beautiful being, with long green hair and a sweet smile.

"Who has called me?" the being said. "Who has said that I don't exist? Here I am, the fairy Hope; maybe someone here needs me."

Gabriel's heart beat like a drum and his legs began to tingle. He suddenly felt a huge desire to ask the fairy to dance. . . and who knows? Maybe to tell her he loved her. But how could he do it?

"Will no one invite me to dance, then?" Poor fairy Hope, what a disappointment! But at that point Gabriel's legs decided all by themselves to straighten up and skip onto the dance floor.

He spun and twirled with Hope all night long and never left her again.

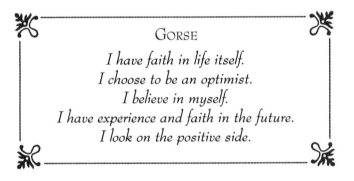

GORSE

I have faith in life itself.
I choose to be an optimist.
I believe in myself.
I have experience and faith in the future.
I look on the positive side.

HEATHER

Do they say I talk about myself too much?
How can they? As soon as I start to speak, they go
away! Sure, I want to be the center of attention.
I want to be cuddled and understood,
and if I'm not, I'm unhappy!

This flower is for children needy of adult attention. Egocentric, they are always trying to draw attention to themselves, not from egotism, but from necessity. They shouldn't be made to feel guilty about this. A need is not a whim; the important thing is to understand and satisfy it.

Heather children are talkative but do not listen to others; they are hyperactive and often hypochondriac as well, since they will get sick in order to be noticed. Sometimes food is the most direct way to blackmail the rest of the family. They may either refuse to eat or gorge themselves greedily, filling up their emotional holes with sweets, a poor substitute for affection.

These children can tire us out, wear us down, and drain our energy, but this is only one more demonstration of their craving for affection. We must nourish them richly with love, as neediness of this kind is carried on through adulthood. Theirs is a condition that should be kept well under control.

Of course, it's easy and tempting to deny that a child lacks affection. But a little honest reflection will show us whether this is true or not. Perhaps we, too, could use a little Heather; if our cup is empty, we can't slake anyone's thirst.

In a negative state, Heather children tend to be exhibitionistic and—let's admit it—something of a pain in the neck. When they drink, they gulp and slurp (as opposed to Mimulus children, who drink as delicately as birds); they eat in a sloppy and unseemly way; they are hyperactive in play but then wear out after five minutes. Although they deeply desire companionship, they are generally avoided by their peers because of their need to be the center of attention. They demand all and give nothing. Yet this behavior stems from their feeling of being deprived of something expected and hoped for.

Games of trade and exchange, by which they may learn to respect the needs of others, are good for these children, as are games in which physical affection, caresses, and cuddles, play a large part. Massage of all kinds; blind man's bluff, in which they must recognize others by touch; and jumping up and down on a mattress, with a lot of rolling around and hugging, are all wonderful for them. They should have many friends, to teach them about sharing. After all, in a positive state, Heather children are the greatest of friends: sweet and cheerful optimists in constant pursuit of the joy that is surely their birthright.

Don't ever hesitate to use Heather, which is almost always beneficial, alone or combined with other flowers. Whatever the circumstance, whatever the child's attitude—negative or positive—you will find in him or her a strong desire to be listened to, to be taken seriously. One flower more will do no harm; use this one freely. Of all remedies, Heather lies closest to the heart of childhood. And don't forget your own inner child; she's there, and she's been calling you for years.

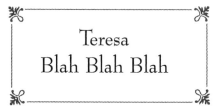

Teresa
Blah Blah Blah

Teresa loved to be in company; she was frightened of being left alone. She liked to chatter on and on and talk about herself, but it was hard for her to listen to her friends. As soon as someone said, "You know, the other day I . . ." she would interrupt and say, "Me, too, blah, blah, blah."

Blah blah today and blah blah tomorrow. Though Teresa needed friends badly, she was gradually left alone more and more, and she wondered why. "How come, when I'm so sociable, everyone's avoiding me? I don't want to spend hours and hours alone like Frances does when she's painting, or like Rose, always embroidering napkins."

The truth was, Teresa didn't contribute much to the group. She needed about as much attention as a newborn, which was a drag, and so she came to be avoided.

The silence that surrounded her was like a nightmare, so one day when she found herself alone in the house, she dialed the horoscope service on the telephone, just to hear a human voice. When it reached her sign, she heard the recorded voice say, "You're not the center of the universe, you know, you're not the only one who exists. Your constant chattering about your problems wears other people down and saps their energy. If you want things to change, you need to learn to listen to the others, and not only that, you have to pull your weight. Stop being such a drag."

"What rubbish," thought Teresa, and she hung up the phone. But afterward, while she was looking for something to do, she heard a little voice that said, "Are you sure that was such rubbish? It seems almost magic to me. That message was aimed directly at you; why don't you listen to it again?"

Who knows where that little voice came from? The fact is that Teresa took its advice, and this time she had to admit that the message was meant just for her.

How strange life is! A simple phone call or two taught Teresa the lesson she needed to learn. These days she's a terrific friend, who contributes a lot to the group and knows how to both listen and help. Once in a while she can even be by herself for a bit—and there's always the telephone!

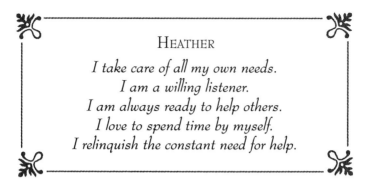

HEATHER

I take care of all my own needs.
I am a willing listener.
I am always ready to help others.
I love to spend time by myself.
I relinquish the constant need for help.

HOLLY

I'm mad, as mad as I can be.
You love my brother more than you love me.
I envy my friends, who are all so much luckier than I am.
Sure I have it in for people!

"This child is really naughty! He breaks everything he touches, he's jealous, and he beats up on his brother!" Actually, he isn't bad, only angry. Hatred, resentment, jealousy, and envy—aren't these emotions with which we're all familiar? No? Think again. When children are quarrelsome, violent, or irascible, when you feel they are being rude and unruly, think back to what might have sparked their reaction.

I recommend the use of Holly whenever a little brother, sister, or cousin is born even if it seems unnecessary, even if the older child loves the newborn very much. Go ahead and use it anyway; it can't do any harm, and may ease unexpressed, or even unconscious, envy.

Holly children are argumentative, never want to apologize, and have a lot of anger to throw around. You can help them by counting aloud from one to thirty together or by joining them in singing an off-color song at the top of your lungs. (Remember, it doesn't take much for something to be off-color at their age.) Have all-out pillow fights or water fights if you can stand it.

During an outburst, it's useless to tell them to stop it and calm down and worse yet to try to get them to be "reasonable." Think instead of what you can do to bring them peace, since deep down the child who needs Holly is screaming, "Help! I want love and I'm not finding it and I'm angry!"

Children with aggressive tendencies should eat very little meat. Even fruit, which creates alcohol in the body, should be eaten only between meals, and only one kind at a time. Give them almonds instead.

If there is a newborn sibling in the house, make sure to set aside special times for your older children, in which they can feel privileged and grown up. She and her daddy might go out for a pizza together, for instance, leaving the baby at home; or you could play a special game with him, bingo or cards, "late" at night when the newborn is sleeping.

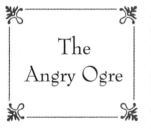

The Angry Ogre

An ogre is an ogre, bad by tradition. Gronco, however, was also enraged; if you were smart you kept your distance. If you got anywhere near him, you were apt to be hit in the head with rocks as big as boulders. So Gronco was generally left alone, and he was angry about that, too. As soon as he caught sight of someone happier than he was, he was eaten up with jealousy and flew into a rage; he would kick, punch, and throw stones at them.

This might have gone on forever, except that one day he happened to ask himself: "What is it that makes me so mad? What is this anger I carry around inside of myself, that makes me feel so violent and bad? Maybe I could be a good ogre. No, what am I saying—ogres are bad, and that's just how it is."

This wasn't true, and Gronco knew it deep down; but in his heart was a big knot of ogreish anger. He tried to think back to when he had started to feel this way. Maybe it was when his sister Gertrude was born, and everyone said what a cute little ogre she was. Or maybe it was that time he had hoped Santa Claus would bring him a gift, and instead he got nothing at all.

Ogres don't cuddle each other or give each other gifts; they're supposed to be bad, and what better way to achieve it? If you look for love and don't find it, it makes you mad—that's how it goes!

Now Gronco began to cry, which surprised him, since ogres never do this. Yet it felt good, it felt as if the tears were washing away all his pain and loosening the knot in his heart. He cried long and hard, and at last he fell asleep and dreamed, and in his dream he saw himself when he was very, very small: Mama Ogre was hugging and caressing him, and singing him sweet lullabies; he was playing with some kittens; and Santa Claus had left a lot of pretty packages beneath the Christmas tree, with a note that said: "To little Gronco, because he is so good!"

When he read these words in his dream he began to cry again, and his tears flowed out into the meadow and gave rise to a thousand colored flowers all around him. Butterflies came close and little birds began to sing. He opened his eyes and smiled at the sweetness of the sight: so much tender beauty just for him. He rubbed his eyes, blew his nose, and began to stroke a lovely little rabbit. At last he was free, free of having to be bad.

He laughed aloud, and said: "All that's missing now is Santa Claus!" And the moment he said it, though it was the fifteenth of July, a sleigh with tinkling bells swooped down from the clouds and brought Gronco all the gifts that he had wanted since he was young.

It felt like a miracle; but miracles do happen, much more often than we think.

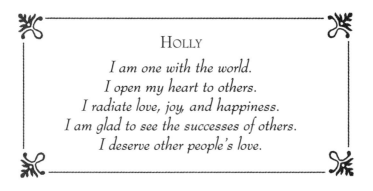

HOLLY

I am one with the world.
I open my heart to others.
I radiate love, joy, and happiness.
I am glad to see the successes of others.
I deserve other people's love.

HONEYSUCKLE

I don't like to leave the house, and I'm so
homesick for my old school! I don't want to grow up, and
I don't want to go to the seashore without my mommy.

Honeysuckle is for children who are homesick, for the first days of school, or for vacations when they want to go home. It is for those who are stuck in the past and refuse to grow. For this reason it is beneficial to children who want *not* to grow up, like Peter Pan. They may be thirteen years old and still go on vacation clutching a teddy bear stained and musty with age.

If they are visiting relatives or going off to camp, give them Honeysuckle to help them enjoy their vacation without suffering from homesickness. This remedy is also useful for adolescents stuck in infantile attitudes and behavior, rebelling against the normal evolutionary process, and for those in boarding schools or in the custody of families other than their own.

What these children need is a sense of continuity. Accustom them to the fact that, although the past is valid and memories are beautiful and important, the here and now is where we live our lives. If you need to help them break a childish habit, like needing a pacifier or a blanket, combine Honeysuckle with Walnut for the transition, so that they may suffer less while breaking the tie.

Make sure that you're not impeding their growth in any way yourself. It's disturbing as well as wonderful to see them mature, but our responsibility as parents, teachers, and caregivers lies in watching them grow up and in letting them go.

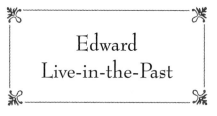

Edward
Live-in-the-Past

Edward lived in the world of yesterday and went around with pictures of himself as a child so that people would say, "Oh, how sweet, what a cute little boy." Meanwhile, Edward wore size twelve shoes; little he was not.

To better succeed in his intention, he made sure that his watch lost time and recorded his movies so that he could watch them backward. He hardly studied so that he wouldn't learn anything new. Even on the train he sat facing the wrong direction because he hoped that by riding backward he could go all the way back to his childhood.

His handful of friends called him Peter Pan because, like the hero of that story, he didn't want to grow up. The difference was that Peter Pan lived through a thousand adventures, while Edward hadn't had a single one.

He spent his days sighing over old photographs and his precious baby bottle and cuddling up with his ragdoll bear, while his classmates were at the ballgame or hiking with the scouts. But he didn't want to go too far from home or from his mother and his things; he didn't want to go forward, only to turn around and go back. It came to the point where he put his shoes on backward and stuck the pages of the calendar back on, under the illusion that he was halting the passage of time.

One day Life passed by those parts and didn't recognize Edward. How could she, when he was always living in the past? Life looked at him curiously and asked, "What are you waiting for? What are you chasing back there? You're not doing anything, you're not even alive. Don't be afraid of the present and future. There's only me, Life—come into my arms!"

Edward hesitated, but a heady perfume was coming from Life.

At first he just savored it; then he threw himself happily into her arms and decided to grow at last.

Like all good stories, this one has a happy ending. Did I say "ending"? For Edward it had just begun.

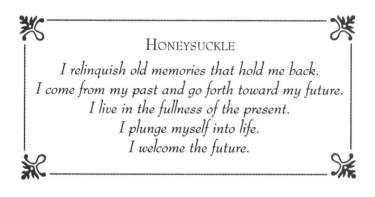

HONEYSUCKLE

I relinquish old memories that hold me back.
I come from my past and go forth toward my future.
I live in the fullness of the present.
I plunge myself into life.
I welcome the future.

HORNBEAM

What a heavy head! Maybe I watched
too much TV or cranked my headphones up too high.
And then there are mornings when I get up and think,
How in the world will I manage it all?

Hornbeam works like a cool, invigorating, and regenerative shower
when children have a hard time just getting up in the morning or
when they act dazed and slow, complaining that their eyes or head
hurts. Hornbeam is also recommended when children are having
trouble finding their own "space" and don't have enough energy
to set any process in motion because they are feeling exhausted.

This remedy is useful for tough times at school, giving a boost
to the mental energy needed to assimilate and carry out schoolwork. Teachers can sprinkle a little in the corners of the school-
room when it seems like the students are avoiding their work or
during the first days after vacation, when the energy level always
needs a lift.

In cases of headache or eye strain caused by excessive TV or
computer watching or if their ears are ringing after hours of listening to hard rock or heavy metal music, compresses of Hornbeam
on cotton laid on their eyes will draw out the tension. In cases of
fever, combine it with Rescue Remedy to ease the feeling of heavi-
ness in the head.

When children complain of a headache, and you know it's because they are tired and overstimulated, don't give them an anal-
gesic right off! Try Rescue Remedy and two drops of Hornbeam,

repeating the dose every five minutes if necessary. It's a good idea to have them lie down in the dark and guide them through a creative visualization (see pages 141–149). If they fall asleep, all the better—it's just what they need.

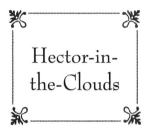

Hector-in-the-Clouds

Just to get up in the morning was a big problem for Hector. Even when he had a full night's sleep, he was still tired and had no desire at all to go to work. A coffee or two, a yawn, and he went, but his head felt heavy. Not even his morning shower managed to revive him. He began to take vitamins to give himself a boost, but with little success—he was still always exhausted.

One day he looked at himself in the mirror and saw that something strange had happened to him: Little clouds of colored smoke were hovering round his head. While he was wondering what kind of weird spell he was under, he looked down and saw that his whole body was covered in these little clouds. They were odd; they took on the shape and look of his face and continued to yawn.

His exhaustion had taken form. It had solidified and now it wouldn't let him do anything at all. Even sitting down and reading or watching TV was too strenuous. With all those little wisps of smoke buzzing around him he felt like he was wrapped in thick cotton batting. What could he do?

Hector tried bathing in foaming seaweed, spraying himself with insecticide, and eating seven ice cubes with lemon juice one right after the other. Nothing happened, but at least the ice cubes were better than the bug spray. He tried sleeping whole days at a time, hoping to rid himself of the clouds, but nothing changed.

One day he decided to resign himself to living with the clouds and he stopped trying to do anything about them. He bought a beautiful mountain bike—he had always wanted one—and took off down the road at top speed. Now, you might not believe this, but those clouds of exhaustion, lazy as they were, just couldn't keep up with Hector, who was pedaling as hard as he could.

So the problem was solved in a flash—with a pair of handlebars and two wheels.

HORNBEAM

I have all the energy I need.
I am strong and complete.
I live my life without stress.
I am fresh and awake.
I take hold of life as I wish.

Impatiens

Good Lord, my friends are so slow,
there's nothing to be done with them! I'm fast,
very fast; I do a million things, one right after the other.
So, once in a while I fall down or bump into things or feel
a little scattered—but I'm fast!

Impatiens children are always in a rush. Nervous and agitated, they do everything in a hurry and are quickly bored. They trip and fall down because they're moving too fast. Pruritis, inflammations, and stomach or bowel spasms are all responsive to Impatiens.

They suffer from all kinds of nervous tics; their rhythm is much swifter than normal. Highly capable, they have trouble adapting themselves to the pace of others. They may be subject to muscle strains and sprains and eat quickly and greedily, without even chewing. Hyperkinetic, never still, their impatience may cause them to stammer, and their hasty way of eating often results in indigestion.

Children in need of this flower are unable to study or play with their peers, being intolerant of tempos slower than their own. They may switch games four times in the course of half an hour. They bump into things and are frequently involved in small domestic accidents.

Clearly, it's no easy task to accustom these children to a calmer pace, but there are games that can teach them to wait their turn and respect the rhythms of others. Help them to appreciate the pleasure of quiet leisure and relaxation by way of creative visualization, in which their active minds may expand while their bodies relax, releasing all tension.

They may also have trouble falling asleep. If so, incorporate a quiet and unvarying ritual into bedtime, one that will help them let go. Slow movement and stretching excercises such as yoga, eurhythmics, and gentle gymnastics are also helpful.

Meditation may sound complicated, but in reality it is easily practiced by even the youngest children. In fact, transcendental meditation, despite its complicated name, can be practiced to great benefit beginning at the age of four.

Children who require Impatiens, in particular, can find real support in meditation. A few minutes each day are enough to relieve the accumulation of stress and accustom them to listen to the silence, to their sensations, to the quiet voice of their bodies.

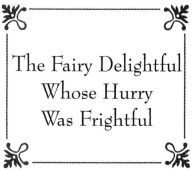

The Fairy Delightful Whose Hurry Was Frightful

As you know, fairies are lively little things. I'm not talking about the ones with wands and pointed caps; I mean those disrespectful creatures with tiny golden wings. Remember Tinkerbell in Peter Pan? That's the kind.

Now, Delightful, besides being that sort of fairy, was also very impatient, always in a big rush. You could never find her with the others when it was time to go and wake up the bluebells; she had already dashed away into the meadow and done half the work. Sometimes she flew so fast that she bumped into trees or mushrooms, so she was always covered in band-aids and bruises.

Delightful fumed when she saw how slow her companions were and preferred to do things herself; no one else could keep up with her. She couldn't understand why anyone would waste time admiring a sunset or a blade of grass sparkling with frost. Even her sleep was restless, and her ways were a little brusque. If another fairy was cleaning a flower's corolla, she would come up and say, "Go on, now, I'll do it. I'm faster than you are, you snail." Since she had no idea how to adapt to the pace of the others, she was usually left alone.

One day, while she was spreading some ointment on her umpteenth bruise, she saw a very large fairy—one of those with the caps—who was slowly threading pearls of dew, one by one, into a necklace. The pearls sparkled so beautifully that Delightful immediately wanted a necklace just like it. She approached the big fairy and asked, "Can I make one, too?"

The fairy answered, "Yes, try. Thread the dewdrops carefully and calmly onto a fine, delicate blade of grass."

"Yes, yes, I understand, I'll do it quickly, I'll do it in a hurry, I'm fast, I want the necklace right away," said Delightful, and in her frenzy she ended up with a fistful of water.

"No, that won't do, little one," said the fairy, "You'll never get your pearls like that. Hurry is bad company, you know. I think you need me."

"Why? Who are you?" asked Delightful.

"I am Patience, and it's time you got to know me."

So a friendship was born. Delightful learned patience, understanding, and a tolerance for others. She found time to appreciate tranquil moments and became kinder and gentler. Now her name really suits her; now she is truly Delightful.

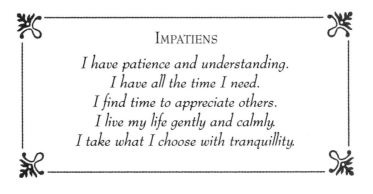

IMPATIENS

I have patience and understanding.
I have all the time I need.
I find time to appreciate others.
I live my life gently and calmly.
I take what I choose with tranquillity.

LARCH

It's useless to try. I'll just never manage.
I'm not like the others; I know from the start that things
will go badly. Things never work out for me, so why should
I even try? I'm sure that tomorrow I'll make a mess of
that essay, as always.

Larch children have no faith in themselves; they feel like losers from the start and so take no risks. They will never take on a part in the school recital or compete in the high jump because they're convinced they can't do it.

This sort of profound discouragement occurs frequently during the school years for a number of reasons. Take care to examine your own negative attitudes about the challenges your children are faced with, as well as those you harbor toward yourselves. If children become accustomed to thinking that things will turn out poorly, they are apt to go from bad to worse. Help them not to program their failures in advance. Larch is an antidote to the sense of failure, so use it whenever you desire success.

Encourage them with lots of positive, affirmative statements (they're free, after all) and involve them in activities devoid of competition and confrontation, ones that bring out their unique skills and creativity: abstract painting, for instance, freeform watercolors or collages put together with paper and found objects.

Positive thinking actually works, so encourage them to throw themselves with confidence into whatever they take on, even the smallest or most seemingly insignificant tasks. It could be a major victory for them just to work the toaster by themselves and serve you the best toast of your life, but only if you allow and encourage them to do so in a completely natural way. It's no problem to keep an unobtrusive eye out to make sure that things go smoothly.

Even in play Larch children must be reassured that all is well and a game is only a game. Entrust them with responsible tasks, authentic ones, not little tricks that end up making them feel like half-wits. Saying to a pupil, "Would you please take care of the roll call for me while I go to the principal's office?" is very different from saying, "How clever you are, you know how to throw the paper right in the wastepaper basket!" Take care not to undermine the self-confidence of these children, since they already live in fear of making a mistake.

Self-confidence is the foundation of any enterprise. Thinking that something will turn out badly means that it probably will. In our society Larch should flow from the faucets, so prevalent is the fear of failure. School, with its system of grades and competitive premise, certainly doesn't help matters. So what can we do?

When we have faith in ourselves, when we realize that we are unique and glorious in our individuality, everything goes more smoothly. Unfortunately, however, we tend to measure ourselves against others. We create overblown expectations that we have no real hope of fulfilling, and so we fall victim to feelings of low self-esteem. In the chapter on Pine (pages 92–95) I have addressed the sense of guilt, which accompanies low self-esteem, that often results from so-called failure.

Larch is particularly helpful in cases of great hesitation and withdrawal. All too often a child in need of this remedy performs poorly in school, and so draws back from trying new things or developing new interests. Don't be deceived by the kind of false self-confidence that manifests as impudence, arrogance, or superiority; you will often find lurking behind it an inferiority complex, masquerading as its exaggerated opposite.

It never hurts to add Larch to other preparations, so it's always better to use it than to leave it on the shelf.

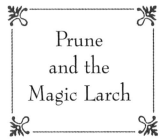

Prune and the Magic Larch

Prune was a gnome. Unlike the others, he didn't compete in the stone-throwing contests—he was afraid that his aim would be off. When they organized an exhibit of drawings on leaves, he was so sure he'd look like a fool that he refused to draw. In the evenings when they danced in the woods, he stayed seated; when they sang, he kept his mouth shut; he wouldn't even play bingo, he was so certain of losing!

He didn't have much fun in life, to say the least, since he was afraid to take risks or try anything new. Even the things he had to do turned out badly, because that's just what he expected: "So, now I have to go out and cut wood—either my hatchet will break or it will start raining." His prediction would always come true, of course, since planning to fail is the surest way in the world to make it happen.

When he went out hunting for strawberries, he was convinced that the ones he found would be rotten. So he hung back and waited till the rest of the gnomes had gathered all theirs—and guess what? The ones that were left were all rotten!

"I knew it, I knew it," he'd whine, and go home hanging his head. But did he decide to go gathering earlier in the day next time? No, he decided not to hunt strawberries ever again.

One day in the forest they organized a flyball tournament, a wonderful game that only gnomes know how to play. Prune really excelled at this game and was especially good at the "hand over hump," a winning move that earned one hundred points. Still, so as not to risk having to play, he hid himself in the thickest part of the forest and fell asleep under a larch.

Now, this was a magic tree. Not only could its branches read people's thoughts and fears, but they could transform any difficulty into a blessing. It's true that the way they did this was a little strange, a little different. But the fact is, that while Prune lay there sleeping, first he was sprinkled with a shower of cold water; then he was pelted in the head with berries; and lastly, a low, very flexible branch gave him a whack down low on his back, that is to say, a kick in the pants!

This ancient formula for instilling self-confidence was known only to the larch. Don't ask me why it was so provocative. I don't know the answer to that anymore than I know how to play flyball. But Prune returned to the tournament and won eight hundred points of "hand over hump"—and that's enough for me. How about you?

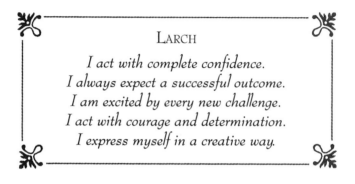

LARCH

I act with complete confidence.
I always expect a successful outcome.
I am excited by every new challenge.
I act with courage and determination.
I express myself in a creative way.

MIMULUS

I feel so shy and I'm afraid of so many things!
I get sick a lot and loud noises scare me. I'm allergic to
flowers and all kinds of animals, and sometimes
I have trouble breathing.

Mimulus is a very useful remedy for all fears of known origin—cats, airplanes, or the dentist, for instance—and for shy, insecure children who hide, blush easily, and hate loud noises and strong smells. These children drink in tiny sips, dislike tasting anything new, and are uncomfortable in company because they don't feel up to par. Although children in need of this flower are generally timid, it is also useful to those who, far from shy, are simply frightened by a particular situation or confrontation.

Mimulus can relieve stammering caused by excessive timidity and other somatic manifestations, to which these children are frequently prone. Mimulus children may develop a stomachache, for instance, if they are caught in a storm, catch a cold after swimming lessons, or suffer an asthma attack in response to familial stress. Fear unleashes an infinite variety of pathologies.

For this reason, Mimulus children are often sick and their convalescence long; illness, for them, is an escape from confrontation with what scares them. Extremely susceptible, they sweat easily, and if covered with a blanket, will cough and sweat all the more.

I have experimented with Mimulus and found it to be a very successful antidote to allergies. My premise is that the allergen, whether it be pollen or horse hair, is a cause for fear and that this fear is something concrete and material. Therefore Mimulus, combined with Crab Apple and Gentian or Willow, can be an optimum remedy for the prevention of allergic attacks.

Engage Mimulus children in breathing exercises such as blowing up balloons or blowing out candles; blowing bubbles is best of all. Learning to manage their breath without conscious effort can be of great benefit to them. Songs, nursery rhymes, and dances of "magic protection" can help them exorcise their boogeymen. The chanted word "Mimulus, Mimulus, Mimulus," inserted in whatever song they're singing, can act as a powerful verbal talisman.

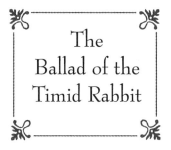

The Ballad of the Timid Rabbit

"Little one, come out with me
and we shall walk upon the lea."
"Mama, no, I must stay in.
I can't go out in all that wind!"
"Leave your burrow in the mountain;
I will take you to the fountain."
"Water frightens me, you know;
lock the door! Don't make me go!"
"The sun is shining overhead;
let's browse around the flower bed."
"Mama, leave me underground,
where no big flies are buzzing round."
"Come to the pond and the good fresh air!"
"What if I find a spider there?"
"Shall we go running in the wood?"
"Too many insects—that's no good!"
"Always hiding down here in your hole—
You haven't been out in a week, all told!"
"I'm so much safer if I stay here.
When I go out, I shake with fear."
"I'm sorry, love, for your own sake,
but Mama's leaving for the lake.
I'm tired of waiting while you hang back;
I'll leave you a salad so you can snack."

"Mama, don't leave me alone in the burrow!"
"Hurry up or I'm off like an arrow!"
"I'm afraid of the lake, just like I said."
"Fine, then, stay right here in bed."
"I'm coming, I'm coming, but I'm so scared.
    There'll be crickets and frogs and toads out there!
    My knees are trembling now with fright,
    just thinking of the awful sight!"
"Take heart, be brave, my little dear;
    Your Mama Rabbit will be near."
"Mother, hold my paw in yours;
    ants are crawling round outdoors;
    and let's be careful near that bush:
    mosquito bites hurt me so much!
    What's that terrible, scary noise?"
"It's only thunder in the skies."
"Run and hide! Here comes the storm!"
"A little rain won't do us harm."
"But now my paws are getting wet!"
"You'll dry off, no need to fret."
"Oh, Mama, I've begun to quake—
    I saw a creature in the lake,
    enormous, with these giant ears
    and teeth that stick out way to here
    and whiskers long and curved as snakes—
    what is that monster in the lake?"
"This is really very funny!
    Look again—that's you, my honey!"

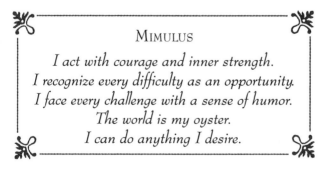

MIMULUS

I act with courage and inner strength.
I recognize every difficulty as an opportunity.
I face every challenge with a sense of humor.
The world is my oyster.
I can do anything I desire.

MUSTARD

*I'm shy, a little ashamed, and embarrassed;
sometimes I blush. I don't talk very much. I'm afraid of
cats and terrified of the elevator. I don't know why I'm so
sad. What do you want me to do? I just don't know! I
feel wrapped up in a big black cloud; I cry and
can't do anything about it. It's awful!*

Even children can sometimes wake up in a black mood. There may be days when they cry and don't know why. Inconsolable, they don't want to listen to reason; and often there is no reason. This may happen during difficult times or in periods of stress, for instance, the week before Christmas. Mustard conquers depression and restores serenity.

Children in frequent need of this flower may live very difficult lives: They may be estranged from their families or be living in poverty, malnourished and inadequately cared for. On the other hand, they may be very wealthy children whose care is entrusted to nannies, religious institutions, or boarding schools, and who lack the warmth of familial affection. In other words, Mustard is for children who are sad. Some of them seem to be wanting for nothing, but what they lack is joy.

Laughter is a tremendous healer. It can loosen the most tangled emotional knots and relieve anxiety and sorrow. When people laugh, their auras are clear and vibrant with color; even their blood flows more strongly throughout their bodies.

In these troubled times the word "joy" sounds absurd and is especially foreign to the regimented world of school. Yet it is simple to live in joy, which works wonders on both children and adults.

Here's a good recipe for joy: Take one smile and spread it around; combine with three bursts of laughter and two silly jokes. Let loose: Roll around in the grass with your children, hug and tickle them, take them by the hand and dance in circles and sing until you're exhausted. Joy itself is impossible to exhaust: It is self-nourishing, growing and growing until it takes over.

You can get addicted to happiness; once you've tasted it, it's hard to do without. Not to worry, though—I've never heard of death by an overdose of joy!

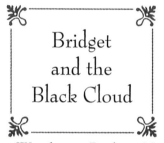

Bridget and the Black Cloud

No one knows why this happened, but one day a strange, thick, black cloud invaded the house of a little girl named Bridget. It settled down on poor Bridget's head and darkened all her thoughts, so that she became sad and began to cry.

Watch out, Bridget! Now it's moving toward your closet, turning all your pretty, brightly colored clothes into a heap of drab gray cloth. Do something quickly to make it stop! You can't live in a gray world, full of tears and sorrow.

Now the black cloud is covering the tape deck; all the tapes begin to play sad songs that make Bridget cry even harder. Can nothing be done to halt this wave of darkness? Pretty soon she'll need a boat to get around in here, because her tears are flooding the room. The walls are damp and gray. Even the tomatoes on the table are turning gray; not even the spaghetti sauce is red anymore!

Stop. Enough! Bridget, make an effort: Try to sing a happy song, or even a stupid one, but sing and dance! Otherwise the black cloud is going to swallow you up.

"Song of sunlight, sung out loud,
Help me banish this black cloud;
Bring me back to joy and color,
Carry off this awful pallor!"

Look, Bridget, your effort has been rewarded. Ray of Sun, Slice of Rainbow, and Lamp of Joy are climbing through your window. In a flash they've dried the room of tears and covered walls, clothes, and tomatoes with brilliant color. The tapes are playing merry music again, and the cloud has dissolved—vanished! Bridget and her friends take hands and dance. Let's join the party! There are pink and yellow candies, cookies covered in frosting, and drinks of every color. Hip, hip, hooray!

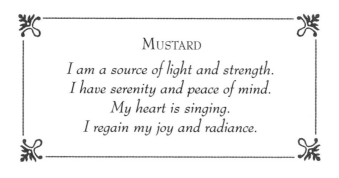

MUSTARD

I am a source of light and strength.
I have serenity and peace of mind.
My heart is singing.
I regain my joy and radiance.

OAK

I'm tired but duty is sacred.
I have to do it all just as well as I can,
even if I get no rest. It's true that I take on other people's
jobs, but someone has to think of these things, and
I'm strong enough to do it.

Oak children keep their noses to the grindstone; they even work hard at play. The concept of rest is foreign to them. They become completely absorbed, throwing themselves into their projects to the point of exhaustion, and then they collapse. They take too much on their shoulders, and then are afraid to renege on all the commitments they've made: schoolwork, ceramics class, tennis lessons, scouts. They feel unable to say, "Today I can't do it; I just can't go." Like oak trees, they weather the storm and hold fast.

They are never, ever absent from school. If they get sick, it is sure to be on a Sunday, when they were planning to go to the lake. Oak can help those students who hit the books so hard that when they go to bed they lie there with their eyes wide open. They are so tired they can't manage to fall asleep, a contradiction in terms that almost all of us have experienced at least once.

We need to teach these hard little workers to relax, to let them know that life is made up of pleasure as well as of duty and that others, too, must do their part. Although all of us are useful, no one is indispensable.

Giving these children Oak won't turn them into idlers or lazybones. It will help them to pace themselves, so that they can enjoy a leisure moment now and then in which to savor their accomplishments.

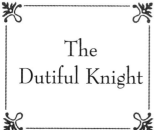

The Dutiful Knight

There was once a knight named Hermes, who was strong and brave and who never rested from his labors. Work was what he knew and work was what he did—hard work, every moment of the day.

The other knights took advantage of him, loading him up with their own jobs and burdens, since they knew he would never refuse them. So he rode from village to village with a huge, heavy pack on his shoulders. Tied to his horse's saddle were more packages, that he was supposed to deliver. He had many other duties as well, which took hours and hours each day, so that he never found time to sleep.

Once in a while he would stop at an inn or lie down under a tree, but he was so tired that he never managed to fall asleep. Instead, he would lie there thinking about the work he still had left to do.

He never complained; quite the contrary. If he happened to see a woodcutter, he got down from his horse to help him. When he finally reached home at the end of the day, did he rest? No, he washed down his horse, cleaned out the stalls, repaired the windows, and went into his woodworking shop to build shelves.

Who was called up to lead all the knights into battle? Hermes. Whom did the king always want at his side in the hunt? Hermes. Who carried the heaviest packages out to the royal carriage? Hermes, of course.

There came a day, however, when his legs refused to go forward, his back felt destroyed, his heart was about to burst, and his nerves screamed: Enough! But Hermes, ignoring it all, forced himself to finish the oaken stool he was making for the queen. When it was perfect and polished to a high shine, he sat down to try it out and fell into a sleep so profound that not even cannons could have woken him up.

He slept a whole day—and a second and a third. When he finally woke, he was crazy with worry. Who had done his work? Why had he been allowed to rest for so long? He looked around and saw that no real damage had been done; everything functioned, even his back and his legs. Then he saw that even resting is a duty one owes to oneself. It's a good thing to work—but not all the time!

OAK

I always let myself rest when I need to.
My rest is profound.
I am open and spontaneous.
I give up struggling so hard.

OLIVE

I'm exhausted; I have no energy at all.
I've been sick and have had a hard time of it.
It's as though my batteries need to be recharged.

Olive is beneficial to sick, disabled, and convalescent children as well as those who are tired or weak and need an energy boost. These children may have drooping or "lazy" eyes, or pupils that tend to roll upward. Polite and well-mannered, they are nonetheless intrinsically sad and expect little good out of life.

Feed them pasta cooked al dente rather than rice, which has a sedative effect. Make sure they eat well and get enough sleep.

Since they are in need of revitalization, don't expect them to throw themselves into activities requiring great energy. Expose them to plenty of sun and fresh air; hug and touch them, envisioning your own energy flowing into them out of your hands.

Combining Olive with Gentian can help them transcend particularly difficult times: Gentian relieves discouragement, while Olive lends strength. For this reason, it's a good idea to add them to the remedy for exams or to use them in conjunction when the family is undergoing stress. In the latter situation, children may have trouble breathing and become very quiet; they exhaust themselves trying to reestablish the harmony they so desperately desire.

Let us instill in our children a love of peace, both individual and universal, which is symbolized by the Olive. These days, when war and racism are dramatic daily realities, the positive thoughts of millions of children could go far to save the earth. Invite the children you care for to light a candle on the first of the year (or any other day) as a symbol of world peace.

Any form of compassion extended toward those who suffer, whether it is effected through money, volunteer work, temporary custody, or adoption, is mutually beneficial. Our own pain tends to assume less importance when we are working to alleviate the suffering of others. Remember that a heartfelt positive thought can help to heal our planet as well as our children.

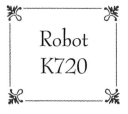

Robot K720

K720 was a robot. He lived in the land of Telemark, and he had plenty to do. Being a robot, he was under the impression that he had to take on all sorts of work, without ever stopping for a moment. He kept the jet-turbine hangars as clean as a whistle, managed the center for statistical data, and taught at the training school, Energetik 45.

Not all the robots worked as hard as K720. They stopped once in a while for maintenance checks—had their electric circuits replaced, their spare batteries recharged, and their push-buttons polished—in other words, they took care to keep in good shape.

K720, on the other hand, never managed to find time to rest; so one day he broke down completely. Not one wave of energy emanated from him. Was he dead? No, but he was so worn down, so totally exhausted, that he didn't even know what was happening. So he went to maintenance and said, "Fill me up, please. Fill me with energy so I can start over." But that wasn't enough, because he was worn out past the point of recovery.

Engineer Bellisario was firm with him. "My very dear friend," he said, "a little fuel and some new batteries are not enough for you. You have to stay here and be completely worked over. Never fear, I'll do it in a hurry and you will be as good as new."

The robot was totally taken apart. He was truly worn out, having abused his capacities without ever stopping to rest. Lucky for

K720, the engineer had all the parts necessary, and so K720 was fixed within a few hours. When he was turned back on, he did feel as good as new; still, he wondered why there was a tag attached with adhesive to his left antenna.

When he asked why, Engineer Bellisario laughed and replied, "Keep that tag on, I put it there on purpose. It says, 'Don't forget tune-ups!' "

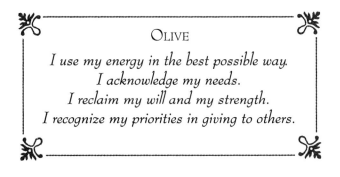

OLIVE

I use my energy in the best possible way.
I acknowledge my needs.
I reclaim my will and my strength.
I recognize my priorities in giving to others.

PINE

I feel inferior and inadequate,
as if I don't deserve what everyone else does.
I'm always saying, "I'm sorry," because I feel like I'm a
bother. I even take the blame for other people's faults.

Guilt! If we could just not pass it on, if we could raise children in the awareness that making a mistake is not the same as being mistaken, we could solve at least half of humanity's problems! Projecting blame and putting ourselves down only generates pain and a sense of inferiority. Use your children's mistakes as opportunities for learning and transformation not as occasions to threaten them with dire consequences or divine retribution. The Creator has better things to do than punish mischievous boys and girls.

I have worked therapeutically for years with the power of positive thought and affirmative speech; there is no way to overemphasize the harm adults can do to children with a careless, or even a well-intentioned but ill-considered, phrase. In my years of work with children, I think I've heard them all. "Look what you did falling down—you broke the stairs! Don't cry or they'll make you pay for them yourself!" "If you keep on this way, you're going to make Mama sick." "Here you have all this food, and children are starving all over the world." "If you don't eat, Daddy will be unhappy." "It's your fault, as usual!"

Children take these rebukes more seriously than we intend them to. They may end up thinking, "My God, what have I done? I must be dangerous." They may even ask themselves, "Why was I born?" Pine is indispensable to children who take on the blame for others, who don't stand up for themselves even when they are right, or who are afraid of having damaged things or people.

As adults, we need to examine and understand our own attitudes about wrongdoing, guilt, and "sin." This is incredibly important, since the physical and psychological manifestations of a misplaced sense of guilt are infinite: aches and pains, grief, migraines, insomnia, inferiority complexes, masochism, contempt for oneself. No one is wholly immune from the need for Pine. Certainly children are not.

We have all grown up with erroneous concepts of what is "sinful" or "wrong." There is a whole different way of perceiving "evil" and "good." Dr. Bach, in his book *Healing with Flowers*, explains this with clarity and grace.

We need to live fully and to understand that error is one of life's teachers. Chestnut Bud, in conjunction with Pine, can help us comprehend this, allowing us to draw upon and work through our experiences, divesting them of guilt.

By freeing ourselves in this way, we can also liberate our children, rather than indelibly imprinting them with guilt, the results of which are ever greater and more complex problems: life lived as a punishment.

Pine is the remedy, and it is we, the parents and caretakers, who should take it first, since we can do nothing until we ourselves are free. Pine should be taken consistently for a long time because the attitudes it is working to reverse are so very longstanding.

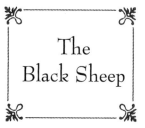

The Black Sheep

Paul was used to being yelled at. Even when he hadn't done a thing, he expected a scolding. Whether he was at home or at school, he always felt somehow to blame, even for the actions of others.

One Sunday his family had planned a trip to the lake, but Paul, unfortunately, came down with a cold, and the trip had to be canceled. When he saw his little sister's and parents' long faces, he felt like a worm. How could he get sick when the boat was there, waiting for them?

Christmas didn't go too well, either. When he was opening presents, he bumped into the manger and three of the little statues fell out; two were broken, and he felt so unhappy about it!

Little by little as things like this happened (the same things, of course, that happen to all of us) he began to feel like the black sheep of every situation. He went around saying, "I'm sorry, I'm sorry." When he called a friend he would say right away, "Am I disturbing you?" When he came to class he said, "Sorry if I'm late," although he never was. On the contrary, he was usually early; he was always trying his best to do even more than he should. Yet it seemed to him that he could never do enough, and he asked nothing in return for himself.

One day he heard on the news that there had been an earthquake. Good heavens! He had drawn a picture of an earthquake only last Tuesday—could this be his fault?

Just then he heard a strange sound—something between a cough and a laugh—and looked up to see a beautiful, shining black sheep standing before him. "Don't worry, Paul," said the sheep, "little boys don't cause earthquakes. What is this ugly word 'fault'? Take it out of your vocabulary! Things happen because they must. Life is like a game of chance: Sometimes you win, sometimes you seem to be losing, but you never know what will happen when you roll the dice. Good and bad are brothers, like black and white.

"Everything is a lesson, and guilt isn't real. If you knock down a vase and break it, you learn the law of gravity. Next time you'll handle a vase with more care. Relax, stop saying, 'I'm sorry,' and know that everything that happens, happens for a reason. We may not always understand it, but it's true. Take a deep breath and start living!"

So that's what Paul did. And the black sheep was gone.

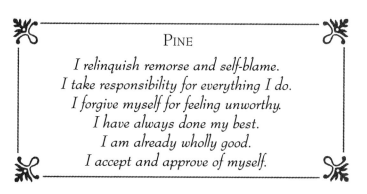

PINE

I relinquish remorse and self-blame.
I take responsibility for everything I do.
I forgive myself for feeling unworthy.
I have always done my best.
I am already wholly good.
I accept and approve of myself.

Red Chestnut

Why in the world is Daddy so late?
Do you think he could have been in an accident?
The two of you will never leave me, will you? What—you
have to take a blood test? Is it serious? Are you really ill?

Children in need of Red Chestnut are chronically anxious. They will ask over and over when their mother is arriving and will start to worry at the slightest delay, asking what can have happened. Even if they know that their mother is always the last to pick them up since she works far away, they will begin to imagine every possible accident that might have befallen her. Their minds are filled with visions of calamity, and it may well be that they have heard too much talk along these lines.

They are so empathetic that they live others' lives as if they were their own and worry less about themselves than about others. Extremely protective of younger children, they may often express a desire for some kind of medicine to render their loved ones invulnerable.

This is the remedy that cuts the umbilical cord—which can remain intact right into adulthood—so combining it with Walnut during weaning can be helpful. In cases of oedipal attachment, it can benefit both mother and son, helping them to gently disentangle and live in peace within their separate identities.

It is very important to teach these children creative visualization. By way of play they can truly send positive energy toward those they wish to protect, disengaging the mechanisms of negative thought that so effectively attract negative situations. (For some examples of creative visualization, see pages 141–149.)

Take care, however, not to trigger off a "savior of the world" complex. Although positive thought is powerful and can go far to better our lives, neither we nor our children should take on exorbitant tasks we have no real hope of fulfilling.

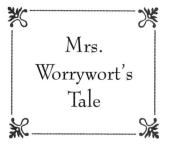

Mrs. Worrywort's Tale

Mrs. Worrywort was always distressed. It wasn't herself she was worried about; it was the others. She wanted everyone safe and secure. If her husband was late coming home, she thought, "Oh, he's been in an accident!" If she saw a child running in the street, she already imagined her under the wheels of a truck. She was forever bundling her nieces and nephews up in sweaters and coats to avoid possible colds.

Every evening the absurd tragedy would begin. "Did I shut off the gas?" Mrs. Worrywort would say. "Louis, come home early from the discotheque. Come home at midnight and not at three, otherwise I'll think that you've been in an accident and I won't get to sleep."

"Mother, they don't start dancing till midnight! It's already ten o'clock. Go to sleep and don't worry and I'll be home by three."

"No, please, that's the worst hour for accidents."

"Mother, is there a best time for accidents? Come on, now, you know I'm a good driver, and I don't drink anything stronger than Coca-Cola."

But she would stay awake in anxious terror until three, imagining doctors and hospitals; and then, since she had so much time in which to think, a little thought about her husband's swollen foot would slip in: "It's probably some very strange disease; they might have to cut off his foot. Oh, if only I could do something!"

But the only thing she managed to do was worry—a lot. If people were paid for worrying, she would have been a millionaire.

Her daughter lived in Canada, so Mrs. Worrywort could tremble at the thought of the cold, of the bears who were surely attacking her child (thirty-five years old, with two children of her own), and of the plane, that dangerous aircraft that was taking them all to Canada to visit at Christmas. Of course, she wanted to see them, but . . . what if the airplane crashed? Who ever knew what would happen?

One day while Mrs. Worrywort was at the hairdresser's, very concerned about not getting home in time to make dinner for Louis (a college graduate, twenty-nine years old), she came across an article in the newspaper that aroused her curiosity. It was about a woman of about her own age who was also always worried about what might happen to her two grown sons. This woman had discovered that if, instead of imagining disasters, she sent thoughts of light and energy in her sons' direction, things turned out very well.

Mrs. Worrywort was perplexed, but she decided to try it—and it worked. That night she sent a ray of light to the disco where Louis was dancing and a ray of light to her husband's foot—and she slept like a baby! And here it was only October; she had two months before Christmas in which to think positive thoughts and send energy over to Canada. Surely the airplane would touch down without any problems—and without any bears!

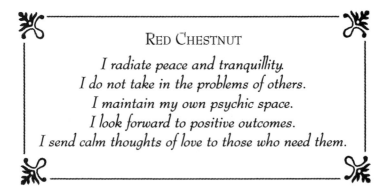

RED CHESTNUT

I radiate peace and tranquillity.
I do not take in the problems of others.
I maintain my own psychic space.
I look forward to positive outcomes.
I send calm thoughts of love to those who need them.

ROCK ROSE

What a panic, tomorrow's the dentist!
What terror, it's almost exam time! I've seen something
terrible, and my poor nerves are shattered.

They are engulfed by terror and panic when something frightening happens, and for them that can be as simple a thing as hearing the tale of Little Red Riding Hood being swallowed by the Big Bad Wolf. Administer Rock Rose to children who suffer from nightmares and nocturnal fears (with Aspen and Mimulus); and in cases of emergency, take it yourselves—along with Rescue Remedy—so as not to transmit your panic to those who are near you. Try not to instill fear in the children you care for by invoking "bad guys" of any kind as punishing agents. Children are not born afraid; it is we who make them so, by saying things whose impact we may not be aware of.

A wonderful way to exorcise fears is to have children draw them. Just seeing their own monsters hung on the wall and being able to compare them to other kids' beasties gives them a way to transcend the fear.

Storytelling and theater are also very liberating. Give them a handful of props and let them work out symbolic dramatizations of fairytales or stories they've invented themselves. You will notice, in these, that good always triumphs over evil. Let them yell out loud when they capture the monster. After all, who can tie up a creature with three heads and exult in a whisper?

Panic is often triggered by arithmetic tests, so start administering Rock Rose the day prior to such an exam. It will help to dissolve the big lump in the throat and slow the fast-beating heart that often precede the problems' dictation. Feel free to add it to the remedy for exams as well, since any test can cause panic. Best of all is to start giving Rock Rose at least two weeks ahead of time until the fateful day, when it can be used as often as every five minutes.

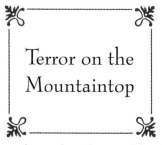

Terror on the Mountaintop

Gilbert was definitely not a timid man: He could cut through the trunks of some trees with a single blow, using an axe so sharp it would make your heart stop. He was a master with both plane and saw. He was strong and he was tough. He wasn't one to flinch at a cut or the sight of some blood; on the contrary, in an emergency he was always first on the scene to help. But one day . . .

One day he and his friend Carl were on the top of a mountain, cutting down an enormous maple. This required strength, precision, and courage, since at the slightest error the tree could come crashing down on their heads instead of falling to earth.

Just as the trunk had been sawn through and the tree was ready to fall, out of nowhere a wild wind whipped up and made the branches of the tree wave about dangerously. Carl didn't realize the danger they were in—that one gust of wind could be fatal—but Gilbert saw what was happening and he was utterly terrified. One extra minute might save them, but the wind blew even more strongly, and Gilbert was afraid that he might frighten his friend into making the wrong move if he shouted. There was not a moment to lose. Suddenly, he remembered how as a child he had been scared of monsters. Now this huge tree with its branches was the monster he must defeat, and he remembered that when he was little he had conquered his fears by singing at the top of his voice.

"I'll try to sing," he thought, "There's nothing else I can do, and at least I'll die singing!"

One note, and one only, burst out of his throat; but that note was so strong that it drove back the wind, and the tree fell safely to the ground. The living force that Gilbert let loose had saved their lives.

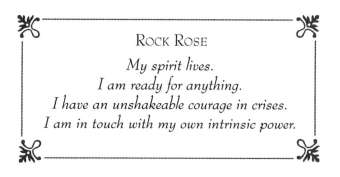

ROCK ROSE

My spirit lives.
I am ready for anything.
I have an unshakeable courage in crises.
I am in touch with my own intrinsic power.

ROCK WATER

I just don't understand the way some people act.
There are ironclad rules to follow, even in eating. If every-
body behaved like me, the world would function much
better. I'm a good role model; I know
how to make sacrifices!

Rock Water is unique in that it is not made from a flower but from water informed with the essence of stone, invoking the image of something granitic and cold. Although this is not a remedy typical to childhood, there are Rock Water children, rigid and perfectionist. If they ask for the mayonnaise, they want it put down in exactly the spot they point out; if their directions are not followed, they won't eat the sandwich because you have violated their inflexible request. Theirs is not a desire for power but the expectation that others will share their own sense of perfectionism. They lack joy and deny themselves pleasure; their drawings are apt to be minimalist and devoid of color.

Rigid belief systems result in difficult lives, characterized by a dangerous resistance to change. To live fully we must be malleable, ready to revise our opinions and go with the flow. Inflexible attitudes are often encountered in children whose families live by unswervable rules, whether religious, moral, or dietary. Such rules reveal an erroneous concept of morality and spirituality and can indicate at times a kind of bigotry expressed through self-restriction. Parents of such families should be the first to avail themselves of the benefits of this remedy, so that they may experience the joyous process of opening to life along with their children.

To overcome the stubborn set of Rock Water children, guide

them toward activities that encourage flow: skating, aerobics, expressionistic dance. There should be no limits, no rules to this sort of play, only the fluid stimulation of their own creativity.

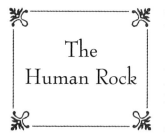

The Human Rock

Constantine never agreed with anyone but himself. He absolutely never made a mistake. It was the others who didn't understand that they were wrong, that he was the perfect example of a human being and a role model for how to live correctly.

Constantine followed a rigid dietary regimen that combined the strictest laws of every philosophy. He never, ever drank a drop of wine, not even at parties; he kept in shape by running each morning at five; he dressed to perfection, with nary a crease or a wrinkle. His every attitude and habit was serious, sober, and composed.

One day, after a bitter argument with his family for reasons he didn't even remember (probably no one wanted to follow the rules he laid down), he became so angry that he stormed out of the house in a fury and sat down in the garden, brooding and muttering and turning things over in his mind. And the more he thought about it, the more convinced he became that he was, as usual, in the right.

When they came out to look for him, his relatives were greatly surprised to find, instead of Constantine, a cold, gray boulder sitting in the garden. But Constantine didn't mind a bit that he had turned into a rock; he liked it, it felt quite pleasant.

Yet as time passed, the peace and quiet began to bore him. A small but nagging doubt assailed him: Maybe his convictions weren't right for everyone, and that was why not everybody shared his own opinions. Perhaps he should have compromised, listened more to the others, but by now it was too late: He was nothing but a big, useless boulder.

Spring arrived and Constantine was covered with beautiful,

brilliant green moss. Flowers of every color sprang up around him and he was content. One day his family came out for a picnic, and as they were merrily eating and drinking, they heard a weak little voice: It was Constantine, asking to speak with them. They were overjoyed and amazed to discover that, instead of lecturing them, he was asking them what they thought about things. He wanted to know their opinions about society, entertainment, fashion, and cooking.

As time went on, they had many interesting conversations, and little by little the boulder began to be able to flex and move. When at last he regained his human form, Constantine was a whole new man.

They threw a huge party and toasted him with champagne. He drank a glass, too, and ate two big slices of cake—and found them awfully, awfully good.

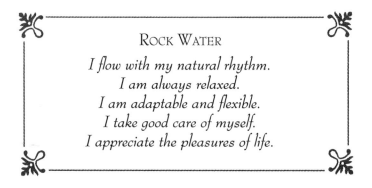

ROCK WATER

I flow with my natural rhythm.
I am always relaxed.
I am adaptable and flexible.
I take good care of myself.
I appreciate the pleasures of life.

SCLERANTHUS

I'm always undecided about things.
I never know which is the right choice. I have sudden
changes of mood, and I never know whether
I'm going to laugh or cry.

Scleranthus is the remedy for ambivalence, for those eternally indecisive children who never know what to choose: "Ice cream or a popsicle? Maybe ice cream. No, a popsicle—or is ice cream better?" It is useful for all alternating conditions: diarrhea followed by constipation, insatiability followed by lack of appetite, tears followed by laughter. It corrects disturbances of equilibrium and other kinetic problems and should be given to children who frequently fall down.

Administer Scleranthus for nausea, vomiting, carsickness (along with Gentian and Rescue Remedy), and seasickness, to which most children are prone. It is also a wonderful remedy for earaches, for children who have trouble balancing when they walk, and for those who pass from laughter to tears at a moment's notice.

It's important for these children to engage in psychomotor activities so that they can learn to coordinate their movements and integrate the mental with the physical. They tend to have problems with lateralization, so activities that help them focus their perceptions precisely are beneficial.

An important key to recognizing the need for Scleranthus is a lack of stability, in the sense that the child in question is living in doubt and indecision and seems not to be "centered" in his or her self. Such children are suffering from a deep disequilibrium that poses continual problems. They are like sails in the wind, meteoric and strongly influenced by the weather. They need to be grounded and centered within themselves.

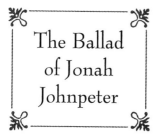

The Ballad of Jonah Johnpeter

This is the story of Jonah Johnpeter,
whose opinions on everything tended to teeter.
His irresolution began with the dawn
when he had to decide which pants to put on:
"Should I wear my green trousers, or should I wear red?
Or should I wear black pants and pink socks instead?
For breakfast should I eat bacon or bread?"
He could pass hours and hours this way,
so that nothing was done by the end of the day.
When vacation time came, he was in great doubt as
to whether to go to the sea or the mountains;
he brought along flippers and rock-climbing boots
and crampons and picks and some old bathing suits.
Eating for Jonah was quite the dilemma:
Pudding or ice cream? Chocolate or lemon?
Pizza or pasta? Sushi or dahl?
Or maybe he shouldn't eat dinner at all?
He bought a camel and a brand-new van,
and he asked the barber for a leg of lamb
because his brain was all askew
from never knowing what to do.
He felt like he was inside-out,
living in eternal doubt.
He couldn't stand any more confusion!
He had to find the right solution!
So he dreamed that he had a scale inside

that weighed and measured and helped him decide;
and when he woke up he saw it was true:
his intuition knew just what to do!

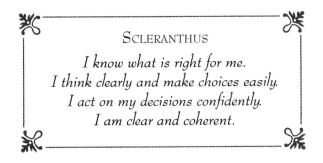

SCLERANTHUS

I know what is right for me.
I think clearly and make choices easily.
I act on my decisions confidently.
I am clear and coherent.

STAR OF BETHLEHEM

What terror—I'm still shaken!
When I was little, something very traumatic
happened to me, and I feel like I'm still there,
like it's still going on.

Star of Bethlehem should be given at birth, the first traumatic experience of every human being. If it is impossible to administer it directly to the newborn, the nursing mother should take it internally and place two drops on her nipples before breastfeeding. Like Walnut, which facilitates change, it is one of the components in Rescue Remedy, itself beneficial during this greatest of transitions in any child's life: from the womb to the outer world.

Practitioners of homeopathy call Star of Bethlehem the "Arnica" of flower therapy because Star of Bethlehem can help with any kind of emotional or physical shock, from an argument with a friend or a violently slammed door to the separation or divorce of a child's parents. Our energetic bodies absorb and retain all sorts of shocks that our minds may forget or not even be aware of. This remedy removes the traces of trauma, whether recent or in the far distant past.

Children in need of this flower may lack energy, courage, or willpower. In order to understand them, it is crucial to get on their wave-length: If their goldfish dies or they see a dead pigeon on the street, they may react strongly and remain distressed far longer than seems normal.

Star of Bethlehem is also commonly used for "unblocking."

Teachers find it useful when otherwise bright students get stuck and can't seem to grasp a new concept, when they are temporarily blocked for some reason. Having obtained parents' permission, the remedy can be administered directly or indirectly, by rubbing some on their hands or sprinkling a bit on their clothes. Little by little you will notice a change in their expression and tone of voice, which will become more lively, joyful, and vivacious.

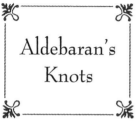

Aldebaran's Knots

Aldebaran was a beautiful horse with a shining coat and a thick, silky mane. One day, however, he was struck down with a mysterious illness that not even the veterinarian could diagnose, and he remained ill for many months.

He nibbled listlessly at his food, and he no longer neighed or galloped as in the old days. Nothing seemed to bring him round—not vitamins, special fodder, or costly syrups. He just seemed to be blocked.

One day an old woman walked into his stall, one of those strange old women you find in fairytales, who appear both foolish and wise. Usually they wear a shawl and carry a basket of magic herbs, but this one, being a modern witch, wore a green and yellow suit and a funny little cap like an airline hostess. She carried a neat suitcase covered in faux fur. There was an absent-minded air about her, but as you know, you can't always trust appearances.

Priscilla, for that was her name, looked at Aldebaran and said, "By all that is strange and wonderful, this beautiful horse needs my help! He has a knot in his throat and a tangle of knots in his belly. Look, look: even his legs are all tied up with strings and ropes, poor thing!" Cecco, Aldebaran's owner, thought the old woman was crazy—what knots and ropes? His horse was sick, it's true, but he would never have dreamed of tying him up.

Then Priscilla turned to Cecco and asked, "Listen, if this is your horse, can you by any chance tell me if he's had a bad fright? If that's the case, I can heal him in a flash."

By now Cecco was convinced that the old woman was truly mad, totally out of her mind. And yet, when he thought back . . . three months before the horse had had a close call; he had almost been run down by the butcher's van. Luckily, nothing had happened; but from that time on, Aldebaran had refused to run or to neigh.

"Well, yes," Cecco said, "Now that you mention it—"

"Say no more," said Priscilla. "It's just as I thought, the terror has tangled him up, hobbled and imprisoned him. A few bites of this herb I have here will heal him instantly."

And that's how it was. Aldebaran ate, and in a flash he was his old self. He threw back his beautiful head and neighed, and then he began to run.

Cecco, who was completely amazed, asked, "What did you give him?"

"Star of Bethlehem," said Priscilla.

"She's definitely mad," thought Cecco, "but she cured my horse."

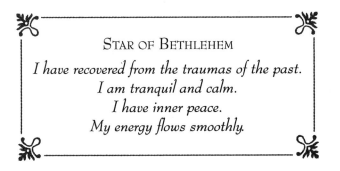

STAR OF BETHLEHEM

I have recovered from the traumas of the past.
I am tranquil and calm.
I have inner peace.
My energy flows smoothly.

SWEET CHESTNUT

I'm consumed by despair and by anguish.
Everyone has abandoned me, I have no hope,
I live in a black hole. . . . What can I do?

In an ideal world you would never have to resort to this remedy, especially for a child. In reality even children, particularly those of school age, sometimes need it after a shocking failure or deep disappointment. They may be living through unbearably difficult times and feel utterly desperate, abandoned by every beneficent force. Or they may be handicapped or gravely ill, struggling with acceptance and wondering if God has forgotten them completely. Don't think for a moment that children can't feel this way; it's often actually worse for them than for adults, since they don't know how to express their despair.

Sweet Chestnut restores joy in life and brings light into the darkness. Meanwhile, do all you can to invest everyday things with joy, so that these unfortunate children may transcend their hopelessness and depression as quickly as possible.

To feel abandoned by God, of course, presumes a certain precedent faith, no matter what you may call the Higher Power: Allah, Cosmos, Buddha, Baba, Great Spirit, or Fate. It is faith in a unique and loving Being, of whom we are an extension and a part. Once we truly understand that divinity lives in us all, there will be no more room for despair.

We will still endure difficulty and suffer sorrow and pain, but by remembering that we are all divine beings, we can perceive our lives with wisdom and live them in joy and in grace. Communicate this to the children you care for, and the vial of Sweet Chestnut need never be opened.

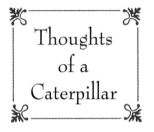

Thoughts of a Caterpillar

"Poor me, what darkness, what darkness in here. How confined I am! Poor me—it was me, I'm the one who shut myself in here and now I have no more hope! Why, why did I do it? The sun, I'll never see the sun again. They told me that afterward I change, but it's not true, there's only the dark and despair here inside and everything hurts me, everything, even my skin. No one can help me, who could even think I'd ever get out of here? It's over, everything's over. They talked about wings and colors, they talked like that to comfort me, but now I feel it: It's death. Yes, I feel bad, I feel like I'm going to explode. Help! Even this safe shell is breaking! Even if it was tight and dark, now it's breaking open and I'm going to die, I know I'm dying! Why? Help! But where am I? The light, so much light, I'm in the open, the colors, the sun, my wings! It's true, then— I'm alive, there is life, there is light, I have wings: I'm a butterfly! I'm flying, I'm flying, I'm alive and I'm flying!"

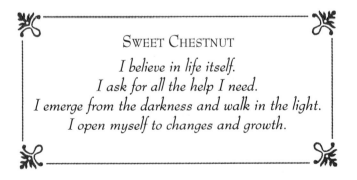

SWEET CHESTNUT

I believe in life itself.
I ask for all the help I need.
I emerge from the darkness and walk in the light.
I open myself to changes and growth.

VERVAIN

*I have so many great ideas,
and I do a lot of good, I think. I really want
my friends to understand and follow my initiative,
but no matter how hard I try, I can't
always convince them.*

Vervain children are enthusiasts, exaggerated in everything they do. They want to involve all their friends in whatever game or sport has taken their fancy and urge them relentlessly to do so. They become so firmly convinced about things that they want everyone else to share their convictions, and if it doesn't happen, they become quite indignant. Hyperactive, they take on a thousand projects but often wear themselves out because they don't know how to channel their energy appropriately.

They may suffer moments of intense disappointment when their ideas are met with a lack of enthusiasm. Their need for followers stems not from a desire to wield power and be "leader" but from a genuine urge to communicate something important. They tend to speak very loudly and walk along stamping their feet like grenadiers; their high-paced rhythm can lead to stress and insomnia. They may eat too much and gobble their food down greedily, since there is a sense of frenzy to everything they do.

These children need to be busy and involved, so entrust them with tasks requiring responsibility. You won't regret it because they are both reliable and indefatigable. They make wonderful scout leaders or volleyball captains, for instance, and are willing organizers of all kinds of games and activities.

What they must learn, however, is how to reserve some of their formidable energy for personal use and how to give themselves and the others some space. Help them to cultivate hobbies and projects they can engage in alone, just for the joy of it, without the need for approval or confirmation from others.

Prince Rudolph

In a country whose name is by now long forgotten, there lived a prince. He was, of course, tall, handsome, and strong, but unlike your run-of-the-mill Prince Charmings, whose only job is to kiss sleeping maidens, Prince Rudolph was bursting with great ideas and wanted to involve everyone in his wonderful enterprises.

One thing he wanted to do was to open a pizza parlor on Mars. Another was to transform the desert into a forest. Wherever war broke out, he arrived on the scene to restore justice and peace (on his terms) and expected his entire court to follow him into the battle.

"Forward, my valiants!" he would shout. And if that didn't work: "Come on, you good-for-nothings!" And if even that didn't rouse them, he would yell, "You low-down ratcatchers, are you going to follow me or not?"

No, Rudolph, they are not coming with you. Try to be a little less impetuous, a little less demanding with your followers; try to understand that not everyone wants to do exactly what you do. If you want to walk all the way to China, fine, do it, but don't expect everyone else to come with you. There are princes who kiss sleeping beauties, princes who go on crusades, and princes who sit in their gardens and think—that's how it should be.

Besides, you have to admit that you're a fanatic. Calm down, stop stressing and straining yourself. These impossible projects will never get done by forcing your friends to participate in them. Yes, you believe in your cause and struggle for your ideals, but if you were less demanding, people might understand better the beautiful things you think about and yearn to accomplish. You can't expect everyone to be just like you. Relax, Prince Rudolph. Follow your heart and let others follow their own.

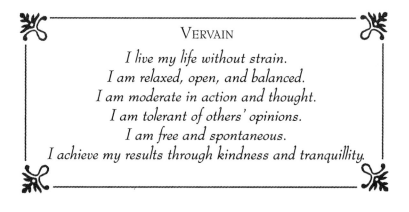

VERVAIN

I live my life without strain.
I am relaxed, open, and balanced.
I am moderate in action and thought.
I am tolerant of others' opinions.
I am free and spontaneous.
I achieve my results through kindness and tranquillity.

VINE

I'm the boss:
Everyone had better do as I say.
I know how to direct operations, and if necessary,
I can be pretty severe!

What little dictators Vine children are! We've allowed them to get away with it and no wonder: It's easier to be their slaves than to create a balanced rapport with them.

When they play, Vine children are always the king or the queen, the father or mother, the gang leader or teacher—in other words, the boss. They order everyone around and exact absolute obedience. There's no arguing with their directives; you do what they want or else.

These young tyrants have few friends (and those they do have are apt to be Centaury) because in the long run other children get tired of being told what to do. Vine children have a violent streak and sometimes resort to their fists to get what they want. They are rigid even on a physical level.

What can you do? First of all, stop granting them all that power. Respect for others is taught by example from day one. Ask yourselves why they have such a negative attitude. Encourage them to engage in improvisation and role-playing, so that they can feel what it's like to be someone else, especially someone in a subordinate position. Last but not least, get them used to taking care of their own basic needs by themselves.

Vine children are spoiled, and that's the truth. Since they were very little, someone has always run to fetch what they want: a teaspoon of this or that from the kitchen, a glass of juice. Once they get used to having a servant at hand, they consider it their birthright. Give them chores that make use of their capacities, but require collaboration with others; don't let them always have the last say.

At Findhorn, in Scotland, there is an "attuning" exercise that coworkers engage in before undertaking any enterprise or making any decision. I highly recommend trying it with the Vine children you care for. Have them take hands, with both their thumbs facing right, so that the right hand is palm-up and the left hand palm-down. Now have them close their eyes and suggest that they feel the beam of light and energy that is passing between them. Keep silent and listen. Then invite the energy to come into the center of the circle. After this exercise you will find the participants of the circle much more disposed to work in harmony, acceptance, and respect with each other.

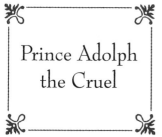

Prince Adolph the Cruel

Prince Rudolph was a fanatic, but he meant well. His cousin Adolph was much worse; he used power for its own sake. No one else had the right to think or speak. He decided things for everyone—and they had better obey. Since he was both cruel and violent, he was greatly hated. If someone didn't obey his orders, that person's head was cut off.

Adolph was ruthless. War was only a pastime to him, a sort of entertainment. He sent many soldiers off to their deaths, while he orchestrated it all. He felt neither sorrow nor pity for all the blood that he caused to flow.

One day during the course of battle, he was unhorsed. Since he was far from the encampment, he sat down under a tree and waited for his soldiers to come get him. But though he waited for a long, long time, no one arrived.

"Whom do you think would come looking for you? Your soldiers are toasting your death at this moment, believing themselves to be free at last of a cruel and wicked tyrant."

Who was speaking? Who would dare address such words to him, Prince Adolph, the terror of the country?

"You can't see me. I'm a voice, and that must suffice for you," it went on. "Know that from now on you will always be alone. In fact, you may just have to stay here forever. As I said before: Who wants you? No one's crazy enough to come looking for you, at least—"

"At least what?" demanded Adolph. "Tell me! I have no intention of staying here to die of cold and hunger. Tell me! That's an order." Silence. "Answer me, I said—it's an order." Another silence, followed by laughter.

"You just don't get it, do you? My dear dictator, you can't give orders to me. Why don't you just rest here a while and give it some thought? Cold and hunger will do you good. They'll give you a glimpse of how much suffering you've caused other people. Bye-bye!"

"No, wait! Who are you? What can I do?" cried Prince Adolph, who, although despotic, was far from stupid.

"Sit and think," replied the voice.

And so he did, for a long, long while. And by the time he was very thin and halfway frozen, he had begun to understand what he had done—never respecting the rights of his people, abusing his power. Instead of preparing himself for kingship, he had only managed to make himself hated.

Then he heard the voice again. "You've come to your senses at last," it said. "Good! Now I'll go call your soldiers. But I'm warning you—you can't see me, but I can see you."

Whose was that small voice? I don't know, and you don't know, either. But King Adolph ruled long and wisely after that, and his name became beloved throughout all the land.

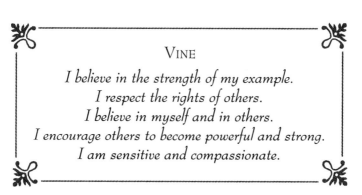

VINE

I believe in the strength of my example.
I respect the rights of others.
I believe in myself and in others.
I encourage others to become powerful and strong.
I am sensitive and compassionate.

WALNUT

I'm moving to a new house and changing schools, too.
I'm not a little kid anymore; I'm turning into
a young adult. All this change is so hard!

Walnut children find transitions particularly difficult because of their ingrained ambivalence. They know what they want to do, but they let other people convince them to let it go.

This remedy should be administered in times of change: teething, weaning (with Red Chestnut), the first days of daycare or elementary school, moving, or going on vacation. It is helpful when children are oversensitive, absorbing and reacting to negative influences in or out of the home, when the people around them are quarreling, for instance. Often in such cases children will develop psychosomatic illnesses to express their unease. This remedy is also beneficial to children of storekeepers or restaurant owners, whose circumstances require them to be in continual contact with strangers.

When you feel the need to protect a child from something intangible that you can't quite explain, even to yourself, administer Walnut, which is a protective agent in that it can form a sort of shield that reinforces the aura and repels negative energies. Creative visualization is also very helpful, both for protection and strengthening of the aura during transitions. Guided meditation can enable the children to envision themselves safe and secure in a new situation. Or you might guide them to visualize a large walnut shell in which they are cradled, rocked and protected, safe from all harm.

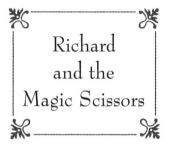

Richard and the Magic Scissors

Ever since he could remember, Richard had been sure that he would do something grand and beautiful with his life. He was fascinated by adventure and longed to go off and explore the most remote places to discover something that was waiting, something only he could bring to light.

But his mother dissuaded him, saying, "Don't leave! I'd have my heart in my mouth if you went far away." And his father grumbled, "You think you're going to find a good job? What adventure? You'll come to a bad end."

So Richard put off his departure and limited himself to short walks in the woods by the house, fantasizing about the future when he would accomplish his great mission. But he was unlucky: On one of his excursions into the forest, he was captured by a wizard who made him his slave. To ensure that Richard couldn't escape, the wizard tied him up with invisible cords, so that although he could work, he could never go beyond the threshold of the garden.

Richard suffered deeply. He, who had wanted to see all the world, was constrained to be a slave and perform the most menial tasks. He was sure that his parents thought he had run away and were now imagining him on Mount Everest or in the jungles of Brazil.

But Richard didn't let himself become depressed. He kept faith with his intuition, which told him, against all odds, that he would one day complete a mission of the greatest importance. With this hope in his heart he carried on, plodding through his days. The cords were very tiresome, but no matter how he pulled and tugged, he couldn't extricate himself. He was under a spell, and only a counterspell could free him.

One night when the moon was full, Richard heard music coming from the garden. The wizard was as deeply asleep as the dead. Richard snuck out and saw hundreds of tiny sparkling fairies dancing in the light of the moon.

"I beg you to help me," he wept, dropping to his knees before them. "I've been held prisoner. Do something for me, I have to escape, I have no time to lose."

The king of the fairies came toward him and said, "We can help you, but are you willing to help us? You see, for many years we have tried to reach the cave of the purple stone, a stone that has the power to give wisdom and goodness to everyone; but it's too far away and we are too small. The climb is very arduous; crags and ravines are a constant danger. The trip is fraught with peril. Are you willing to take this on?"

"My God in heaven, I've been waiting for something like this for a lifetime! Free me and I swear to you that I'll bring back the purple stone at any cost," shouted Richard.

"Ssshhh! Don't wake up the wizard. Here, take these magic silver scissors, and in two or three hours you'll be able to cut the cords. I know you can't see them, but just keep cutting the air around you," said the fairy king.

Richard freed himself in less time than it takes to tell it and ran merrily off on his way. This was the moment he had been waiting for all of his life. The chance to fulfill his dream had been born from the depths of his imprisonment. "Wait, purple stone, I'm on my way!" he sang out, and set off on his great adventure.

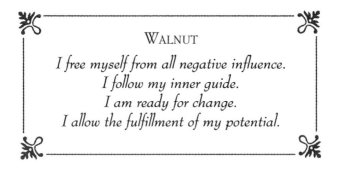

WALNUT

I free myself from all negative influence.
I follow my inner guide.
I am ready for change.
I allow the fulfillment of my potential.

WATER VIOLET

Why should I hang around with those kids?
They're worthless next to me! They say I'm stuck up,
but they always ask my advice. I'm nice, I listen to
them, but I'd never ask them for anything.
It would be useless, and actually
I prefer it this way.

Proud Water Violet children place little trust in others and can come across as haughty and aloof. They are timid at times and dislike leaving the house. Rigid in their judgments and quick to disapprove, they seldom mingle with other children, since they feel themselves to be so superior to them.

Still, these are the children their classsmates call for help with their homework. They impart the needed information politely and then hang up, shaking their heads in wonder and going back to whatever it was they were doing. Water Violet children never ask help from anyone else; they wouldn't lower themselves.

Actually, relationships are their biggest problem. While it's true that they're sought out for advice, they are hardly ideal playmates. They often give the impression of being much more mature than their age, which in fact they are.

They may suffer from respiratory difficulties, given their reluctance to "share the air with others," as well as trouble with their joints as a result of their emotional rigidity. Both these symptoms spring from spiritual imbalance.

Your main task is to try to convince these children to be more childlike. This is no play on words, but the very crux of the problem. It is important to develop their sense of humor. Jokes and laughter and silly games are just what they need to loosen up and enjoy being the children they are.

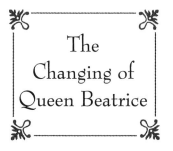

The Changing of Queen Beatrice

Beatrice was not only a beautiful queen but a powerful sorceress as well. She lived in a crystal castle, of which she was fiercely proud, and she hardly ever left it. Instead, her subjects would frequently come to the castle, in search of good advice or some herbal potion for pain. The queen would smile and write them out a prescription or pass on a suggestion, yet her manner was always superior and aloof.

It's not that she was ill-mannered; on the contrary, she was always quite nice, but she never laughed or held out her arms for a hug. She lived in a world completely her own, a world shut off from all others, and she thought this was as it should be. While she never refused her counsel to those who sought it, she would never, ever have lowered herself to ask for help of any kind or even for a little company to while away the time.

Beatrice was alone, and she was lonely, but no one measured up to her standards. There was no one she felt she could share her time or knowledge of magic with.

But one day, as she was strolling by the lakeshore, she came upon a basket in which a little bundle of rags was piteously crying. Drawing back the cloth, she uncovered a beautiful little girl and decided to adopt her. She took her to the castle, named her Caroline, and raised her with care, efficiency, and affection. But Caroline, who never heard a peal of laughter and never had anyone to play hide-and-seek or ring-around-the-rosy with, grew sadder and sadder each day.

Queen Beatrice consulted her magic tomes to find out if there was an herb or decoction that could make her daughter happy, but she discovered that only the company of other children could bring Caroline that kind of joy. So she threw open the castle doors and began to give parties and puppet shows. Not only Caroline but she herself began smiling and laughing.

From that day on the crystal castle was a meeting place for everyone, filled with merriment and peace. Beatrice discovered that, like the other parents, she was as glad to listen to advice as she was eager to give it. They all exchanged recipes and household tips, swapped books, went shopping together, and helped each other to organize birthday parties and holidays.

Beatrice even began to dress more comfortably and less seriously. One day her old aunt, who had dropped in to visit, hardly recognized her niece. The queen, dressed in blue jeans and pink tennis shoes, was pushing little Caroline back and forth on the swing and singing at the top of her lungs. The once austere castle had become a kind of amusement park. Beatrice's aunt, completely thunderstruck, cried out, "This is a miracle!"

And of course it was. There are many miracles, happening all around us, and usually we don't even see them.

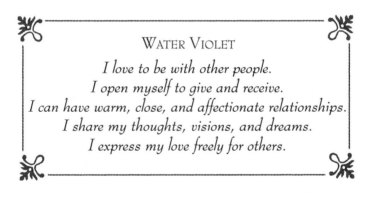

WATER VIOLET

I love to be with other people.
I open myself to give and receive.
I can have warm, close, and affectionate relationships.
I share my thoughts, visions, and dreams.
I express my love freely for others.

WHITE CHESTNUT

It feels like my head is always filled to bursting.
I can't seem to relax because I can't get away from these
fixed thoughts. It's not like I ask for them;
they just appear and there's not a thing
I can do about them.

White Chestnut children have fixed ideas; from the moment they wake up to the moment they fall asleep they may be obsessed by thoughts from which there seems no escape. Their minds are always at work, never relaxed. These children may be repetitive because they are unable to break free of whatever is going round and round in their heads (unlike Chestnut Bud children, who find it hard to learn). For this reason, they may appear disconnected. They may tire easily and suffer fiercely from headaches.

Try to discover the reasons for their fixations and do what you can to diffuse them. Star of Bethlehem may also be needed if their condition is due to a past but unresolved trauma.

Often adults are unwitting causes of children's unease. As always, I recommend that you examine your own attitudes and behavior to see if your convictions and actions—or even careless comments—are causing the child you care for discomfort or confusion.

White Chestnut children can benefit greatly from relaxation exercises and from liberating, creative activities in which touch and the manipulation of materials help to disengage them from their mental obsessions. Sculpting with playdough can be a cathartic activity for them. Make it together (see the recipe below) and watch how these simple and natural ingredients are magically transformed into a malleable and brightly colored dough.

Sometimes we limit our imaginations by buying premade toys when preparing them ourselves is both satisfying and considerably cheaper. The simplest household ingredients can become creative material. Food coloring, for example, makes absolutely wonderful watercolor paint. Just mix a few drops (the color is highly concentrated) of red, blue, green, or yellow food coloring with a little water in very small jam jars, and hand the artist a brush. Like homemade playdough, these watercolors will last indefinitely and cost almost nothing to make.

Recipe for Playdough

> 4 cups of white flour
> 4 cups of water
> 2 cups of fine salt
> 4 teaspoons of almond oil
> 2 teaspoons of cream of tartar
> Food coloring optional

Mix all the above ingredients (except food coloring) thoroughly in a pot until the mixture is no longer lumpy. Cook over a low flame for about five minutes or until the paste no longer sticks to the sides of the pot. Add food coloring if desired. Let cool, knead well, and play. To save the dough, store in an airtight container. To dry and set the sculptures, leave them out to harden.

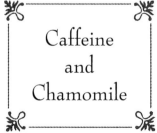

Caffeine and Chamomile

Caffeine worked for the data bureau, and Chamomile worked for the agency of endowments. They both held positions of great responsibility, and their work was very demanding.

Caffeine ran around all day without a break—cellular telephone, secretary, three cups of coffee and a cigarette, and then he was rushing off to the airport. What stress! His brain was a whirlwind of conflicting ideas and thoughts. A wizard would have been able to see lightning flashes and thunderbolts zipping around Caffeine's head.

The same wizard, looking at Chamomile, would have seen only a beautiful rainbow. He worked hard, too, but at times he sat very still with his eyes closed, and if you asked him what he was doing, he'd say, "I'm meditating, relaxing my mind and recharging my energy."

Caffeine thought his colleague very odd and said to himself, "He's off his nut, out of his mind!" Still, he had to admit that Chamomile was always smiling and serene, yet managed to get all his work done on time. In fact, the agency of endowments had a much higher output than the data bureau run by Caffeine—that was the strangest thing about it.

"Listen, Chamomile," he asked him one day, "when you're over here, I mean, all that stuff that you do, well, what I want to ask is, what do you mean when you say you're relaxing? I don't even relax when I go to bed at night. Don't you worry, don't you think about your work?"

"Of course I think—I have a brain, don't I? But I direct my thoughts, I don't let them control me."

"Ah, excuse me, I don't think I understand what you're saying."

"I'll give you an example," said Chamomile. "Think about being at the wheel of your car: Do you drive it or do you let it drive you? So, I drive my mind and my thoughts; I don't let them get out of control and go off the road."

Caffeine was disconcerted, but the example was a perfect one. He had a huge, fancy car.

"Listen, Chamomile," he said, "I'm sorry if I'm bothering you."

"Don't worry, you're not bothering me. I'm fine, no one ever annoys me."

"Well, then, here's the thing, do you think that—no, maybe not, I don't know—you know how it is—well, what I meant to say was—"

"I understand," said Chamomile, with a smile. "You want to

know if you can learn how to relax, too, isn't that right?"

"Right." Maybe Chamomile wasn't so far out after all. "You got it right away."

"It's because of these meditation techniques. And the answer is yes—even a child can do what I do. It's extremely simple: All you have to do is desire to change and decide that you prefer a relaxed life to a life of stress. If you want, I'll explain how it's done."

"Great, thanks! Should we talk over coffee? Or maybe a cup of chamomile tea would be better."

"Come on, I'll explain it over a cup of tea."

Congratulations, Caffeine! Soon there will be a rainbow around your head, too!

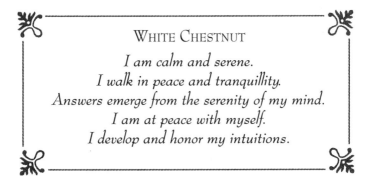

WHITE CHESTNUT

I am calm and serene.
I walk in peace and tranquillity.
Answers emerge from the serenity of my mind.
I am at peace with myself.
I develop and honor my intuitions.

WILD OAT

What will I do when I get out of school?
Good heavens, who knows? Yes, there are things that
I'm good at, but it's so difficult to choose. It's not that
nothing satisfies me; it's just that I'm so uncertain.

Never content because they don't know what they want to do,
Wild Oat children are chronically dissatisfied, lethargic, and bring
very little to conclusion. They may undereat for lack of interest or
overeat to fill the gap left by their great dissatisfaction. Use this
remedy with children who appear uninterested, when in reality
they are disoriented, and with those who passively accept situations that they would do better to take charge of.

Wild Oat can greatly benefit teenagers facing a daunting variety of choices. Who knows exactly what one wants to do at the
age of fourteen? Yet school (and life) move on, and Wild Oat can
help to clarify otherwise latent capacities and desires.

Wild Oat children may experience problems with the thyroid—
the organ most linked to creativity—so introduce them to the
most varied and creative activities you can think of. Games and
activities in which purposeful choice is the determining factor
can help them comprehend the importance of personal power in
its most basic and loveliest sense: the magic "I can." The choice,
however, should be theirs. Your job is to encourage them, to emphasize how capable and "together" they are.

Wild Oat is deeply connected to the principle of creativity,
which embraces much more than the arts. We tend to limit it in

this way, but creativity is the art of life: It is finding purpose, pleasure, and joy in all that we do. When defined in this way, just setting the table or reorganizing the drawers can be a creative act.

A few days ago I heard a story I'd like to pass on, since it so beautifully illustrates this point:

Three men were working side by side, cutting and transporting stones, when a fourth person approached them and asked them what they were doing. The first man swore and cursed the lot that had led him to toil and sweat like a beast for three miserable coins. The second said he was working to keep his family in food, but when he went home in the evening he felt happy and no longer tired. The third man was singing, cutting, and carrying the stones as if he were dancing, and said with a radiant smile, "I'm building a temple for my Father!"

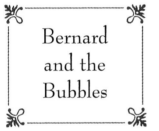

Bernard and the Bubbles

Ever since he was little, Bernard would sigh, "If only I could play basketball," but he stayed at home instead to watch the games on his TV. He would say, "I sure would like to play the guitar," and put on a record. He had many aspirations but lacked the will to put them to the test. He wanted to go to college but couldn't seem to choose a school and ended up working instead at a job he didn't much like.

Deeply dissatisfied with his life, he seemed to be living inside a sack. He had put himself there but couldn't seem to climb out. For instance, if he wanted to take a trip, he would pore over maps and tour brochures and stay at home, sighing, "Oh, if only I could. . . ." All his friends had hobbies. Once he bought materials to build a pantry with but never even built a single shelf. Every day he watched a TV show called "Fishing Today," but he didn't know a fishhook from a lure. Instead of biking around the countryside, he put a stationary bicycle in his bedroom. An art book stood in for paints and brushes. He had a shelf full of cookbooks and loved to read the recipes, but he never tried to make one.

Bernard found the courage to admit that he was dissatisfied and felt deprived, but what was keeping him from doing as he pleased? Only his passivity; he had no one to blame but his own lazy self.

Finally, one day a fairy took pity on him and came to his aid: She put some magic drops in his water. They turned into countless sparkling bubbles, and when Bernard raised his glass and drank, he felt a shiver run right through him and said, "You know what I'm going to do? I'm going to go out and buy a red bike and a backpack and take off for the mountains, and I'm going to gather wildflowers and start a dried flower collection, and when I come back I'm going to get brushes and paints so that I can paint them, and then, and then—"

He joined a basketball team. He booked a flight for England and learned to play the guitar. He went out fishing and caught some trout as big, in fact, as Bernard's own potential, which he was finally exploring. By a stroke of luck the fairy had come just in time, and her bubbles had woken him up.

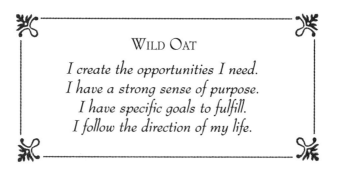

WILD OAT

I create the opportunities I need.
I have a strong sense of purpose.
I have specific goals to fulfill.
I follow the direction of my life.

WILD ROSE

What a drag!
I mean, what am I supposed to be doing?
I watch television, take a nap or two, but I don't seem
to want to do much of anything, really. I'm tired,
everything's such a bore.
Oh well, what can you do?

Apathetic, tired, listless, often without appetite, Wild Rose children tend to be pale and appear sick. They need help developing the energy and interest required by the lives that await them. Convalescent or resigned to their situations, they never get angry, but nothing excites them.

They spend hours in front of the TV, but not with the fervid curiosity typical of childhood; instead, they vegetate, hypnotizing themselves with ads and cartoons. They are lacking in willpower, limp, sad, and drowsy.

To restore life to such children, try to nourish your own energetic potential so that you can communicate the will to live to them. In addition, try to understand what might have caused them to develop such a pervasive feeling of sadness.

They may just be suffering through some transitional phase, as in convalescence. Your job is to find the key that will set back in motion their desire to do things and, above all, their desire to *be*. It doesn't matter what the key is: It could be collecting bottle tops or cutting pictures out of magazines to make a collage. The important thing is to keep the energy level high.

Engage them in lively activities. Merriment, laughter, plenty of stimulating food—even a little chocolate spread, scooped from the jar with a finger (which we all know makes it taste better)—along with administration of Wild Rose, will spark these children's energy and bring them back to the sheer joy of living.

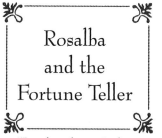

Rosalba and the Fortune Teller

When Rosalba woke up in the morning, she was already tired. What a drag it was to do the housework every day! She'd make a quick swipe here and there and then plunk herself down in front of the TV and watch the soap operas for hours.

"Lucky them," she would say to herself, "My life is so boring, and they have it so good," without ever reflecting that what she was watching was fiction and not real life at all.

Aside from that she didn't do anything, since nothing interested her. Her neighbors had invited her more than once to go with them to the gym or join them for a walk around town, but she was always too tired to go. Besides, what a complete bore it would be to work out at the gym or play bridge!

One of her neighbors was always singing as she did her housework, and Rosalba just couldn't understand it. No more did she understand her cousin, who tried out a new recipe every day—how tiring! Rosalba herself munched on the same old pasta with butter each evening, which was a drag, of course. But it didn't require much effort.

One day on one of the soap operas the heroine went to a fortune-teller to have her future read:

"Long trips to foreign lands, luck in love, and honor! You will become rich and famous: I see swimming pools and servants, furs and jewels, masses of red roses, and exquisite goblets of champagne," said a rather funny actress, draped in necklaces and wearing long, dangling earrings. A multicolored turban was wound around her head, and she sat in a little room crammed with amulets and talismans.

"That's it!" thought Rosalba. "I'll go to a fortune-teller and have my cards read. Who knows? There may be something wonderful in my future!"

So she went to Madam Cesira, of whom everyone had said, "She's great, she sees you just as you are," but when she got there, she was rather disappointed. Madam Cesira did not wear a turban, full skirts, and dangling earrings; she was dressed in a very ordinary skirt and blue jacket. Nonetheless, Rosalba was anxious to hear her fate, so she went in. There were cards on a table but no owls or amulets around, only furniture and pictures. It was a very normal room.

"Dearest Rosalba," said Madam Cesira, "have you come to find out your fortune? Know, then, that we create our own destinies. Right now all I see around you are soap operas and an aura of boredom—did you expect to hear something that doesn't exist? The truth is that your life is tiresome because you yourself are tiresome and apathetic. You don't interest yourself in anything; you do as little as you can get away with, and even then without the slightest enthusiasm. I know that you'll get up now and go out slamming the door because you hoped to hear me predict Prince Charmings and champagne, but that's not how it goes."

Rosalba got up and left, slamming the door just as hard as she could.

The fortune-teller laughed and said to herself, "I'm pretty good—she did just what I predicted! Poor Rosalba, who knows if she understood a word I said? I wanted to help her, but she didn't even pay me . . . ah, well." Still chuckling, she took up her knitting (she was making a sweater for her daughter).

And she was right: Rosalba had understood nothing. She was resigned to a tedious life; nothing stirred her interest or excitement. It was all a drag, a terrible bore.

And isn't it a shame? If she had listened to the truth and faced it, she might have changed, freed herself from her torpor, and begun to really live. The choice was hers. For Madam Cesira was right: It is we ourselves who create our fates.

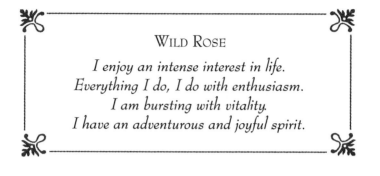

WILD ROSE

I enjoy an intense interest in life.
Everything I do, I do with enthusiasm.
I am bursting with vitality.
I have an adventurous and joyful spirit.

WILLOW

*Everything bad happens to me, I'm the unluckiest person
in the world. Everyone else is having such a good time,
but they'll find out how it is someday, and I'll be glad of
it! Then they'll know how it feels to be me— miserable,
misunderstood, and unlucky.*

It's a sad thing when children are already pessimists. Before even
tasting the melon, Willow children know they won't like it. They
get onto the merry-go-round already convinced that it's a swindle.
Their very attitude attracts disappointment, since that is what
they expect.

Willow children also hold grudges, often for a very long time,
so that when something goes wrong for a friend, they rejoice. If
some schoolmate has done badly on an essay, for instance, they
are deeply satisfied and think, "That'll teach him! I'm always getting bad grades—now it's his turn, let him see how it feels!"

The teacher, the principal, the scout leader, and coach all "have
it in" for them. Poor defenseless victims, nothing is ever their
fault; it's either someone else's fault or plain bad luck. They tend
to take refuge in illness, to demonstrate to the world (and specifically to their family) that they are wretchedly miserable and need
sympathy and consolation.

Although they whine and complain that nothing ever goes right,
they don't understand that they are responsible for the situations
they find themselves in. Needless to say, they don't have many
friends. Who wants a friend who's whiny, pessimistic, vindictive,
and a real pain in the neck?

Willow children need to learn that they are not victims, not unlucky. They must be taught that negative expectations create negative situations. Do whatever you can to show them that optimism beats pessimism; that having fun beats complaining; and that positive thinking brings good things their way. As usual, I also suggest that you explore all the possible causes for their feelings of victimization. And of course, administer Willow.

A little applied psychology can be helpful. If, for instance, you're choosing whom to send down to the courtyard to gather some leaves for the class collage, and you see that your Willow child's expression is already dark and resigned, choose her for the mission and watch that expression change. How quickly her desire to participate in the project will revive! Or if you're playing a board game, checkers, or cards, you might consider a little innocent cheating once in a while, so that he gets to win. A trick or two is admissable when it is to such good purpose!

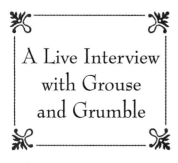

A Live Interview
with Grouse
and Grumble

"Gentlemen, thank you for agreeing to this interview. We know that you're brothers and come from the country of Nothingevergoeswellforme and that you believe in bad luck. Is that correct?"

"Yes, indeed, we're the two unluckiest people in the world, isn't that right, Grouse?"

"It's worse than that, Grumble. We're victims; nobody loves us, in fact, everyone hates us."

"Are you quite sure of that? At any rate, tell us something about yourselves. Who are your friends, for instance? What do you enjoy doing together?"

"Well, to begin with, we don't care for friends very much, and anyway, no one ever comes to visit us. They say our coffee is too bitter, but that's how we like it. They can fend for themselves, you know; we're not about to change for them. They're all disagreeable, lazy egotists, anyway."

"You're absolutely right, Grouse. I'm delighted, for instance, that a brick fell on John Glad's foot; maybe now he'll stop laughing and simpering like the idiot that he is. God only knows what he finds to laugh and be happy about, anyway; he doesn't have a very good job. While we, of course—but, you know, we have never, not even once, won the lottery!"

"So you two play the lottery a lot?"

"No, what's that got to do with it? We just never win."

"But if you don't play—"

"Listen here, young lady, don't you go lecturing us! We know how unlucky we are and how badly the world treats us, don't we, Grumble?"

"Certainly, brother, even our garden's no good: By the time the tomatoes ripen they're full of worms, the apples grow gray instead of red, and even the lettuce comes up limp and white. And if you must know, it's all the fault of that neighbor of ours who plays the radio so high it's blasting. All that music kills the lettuce."

"Really? I always heard that plants love music."

"My eye, plants love music! I'd like to plant one on all their behinds, kick 'em out once and for all, got that?"

"Please don't get mad, but you seem to me to be pessimists— you see everything in a negative light."

"Grumble, I warned you not to accept an interview with this woman. I knew from the start it was a stupid thing to do, but you, you're just too good, and now all she does is criticize us. See? Great reward! It's just another rip-off!"

"No, excuse me, but what are you talking about? What rip-off? We paid for your trip and hotel."

"Speaking of that hotel, it's a real dump! You can't even see the garden from our window—all you can see is an old dilapidated wall full of broken-down bricks. It's disgusting!"

"That's the Colosseum!"

"Maybe so, but I would have preferred a garden—how about you, Grouse?"

"Look, I would have preferred to stay at home. This morning they hardly gave me a crumb: just brioche, buttered rolls, café au lait, cookies, marmalade, honey, and orange juice—what the devil kind of breakfast is that?"

"All right, could you explain to our audience the reason you feel you're so unfortunate?"

"It's just everything. Everything always goes wrong for us and it always will, won't it, Grumble?"

"That's understating it, it's much worse than that, Grouse. You're too much of an optimist, you always have been."

"We interrupt this transmission for technical reasons . . . ."

"You see? We were right! Everything breaks down, goes wrong, turns out badly for us—that's life!"

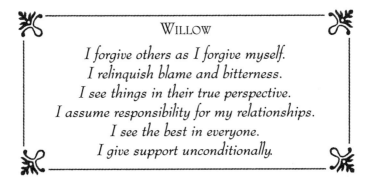

WILLOW

I forgive others as I forgive myself.
I relinquish blame and bitterness.
I see things in their true perspective.
I assume responsibility for my relationships.
I see the best in everyone.
I give support unconditionally.

THREE CREATIVE VISUALIZATIONS

In this section you will find three examples of guided meditation, or creative visualization, that I have found to be very successful in working with children. They are meant as guidelines only, as a jumpstart for your own imaginations. Infinite possibilities unfold within the course of these exercises. Don't hesitate to be spontaneous and let your inner voice direct you through the journeys you are sharing. Never rush; the pace should be slow enough and the pauses long enough to allow each child's unique inner visualization to flower to fulfillment.

Visualization for Relaxation

Children, lie down and get comfortable. Don't cross your arms or legs. Hold them a little apart, nice and loosely, and relax. Now close your eyes gently—don't squeeze them—and get ready for a wonderful game of imagination: We are about to enter the magic world of colors.

Let's take three deep breaths together, deep and slow . . . that's right. Now let the tension seep right out of all your muscles so that they become very limp and soft and loose. With every breath your body is softer, looser, and more relaxed.

Now imagine a rainbow like a bridge onto which you can climb into heaven, passing through all the colors. Walk through red and enjoy how strong, healthy, and vibrant you feel. Now enter orange and let it wash through you, leaving you calm and serene. From orange pass into yellow, and notice how clear your mind is and how lovely and peaceful all your thoughts have become. Now you find yourself in green and feel at peace with everything and everyone, tranquil and relaxed. From green pass into blue, beautiful blue washing through you, letting you know how much you love yourself, your very own self, the splendid child that you are. Open up and let yourself feel the love you have for yourself and for everyone else in the world. Now walk forward into indigo and look inside yourself. You will find a little secret spot where all that is best and most beautiful in you lives—that is your heart. From indigo pass into violet and feel the great strength of that beauty inside you, and know that you yourself are creating all this.

Stay completely relaxed. You are now standing on top of the rainbow with clouds all around you. Spread your arms and get ready to fly, which you can do as easily as you breathe. Launch yourself off the rainbow and fly up and up and up, and keep your eyes on the distant sky. You will see that someone is approaching you and holding out their hand. I don't know who or what it is, whether it's someone you know, a person you've never seen before, an animal . . . only you can see the lovely being coming toward you, to keep you company in this magic world. If you don't know this being, ask its name.

Take your guide by the hand and go flying together. What do you see, whom do you meet? It may be that you pass out of the clouds to some other beautiful place that you like very much. Look all around and listen to all the sounds; touch anything you want; play with your friend.

Now I'm going to stop talking for a few minutes and let this soft, sweet music guide you along on your journey. . . . When you hear my voice again it will be inviting you to come back and, if you like, tell the story of your beautiful experience.

Now say goodbye to your friend, your wonderful guide, but know that anytime you want, you can call on that being and it will come to help you and keep you company.

You are standing on top of the rainbow again. Begin walking backward through all the colors: violet . . . indigo . . . blue . . . green . . . yellow . . . orange . . . red. . . . Open your eyes slowly when you are ready and notice how good you feel.

Visualization to
Reinforce the Aura

Lie down and get comfortable. Don't cross your legs or your arms. Close your eyes and relax completely; let all your muscles go soft and loose. Now take three slow, deep breaths . . . one . . . two . . . three . . . and three more . . . one . . . two . . . three. . . .

Place both your hands on your solar plexus, which is about where your stomach is. Now, without opening your eyes, look around and you will find yourself in a wonderful room, the most beautiful room you have ever seen, made all out of gold. Look down at your own solar plexus and notice that it is now covered by a great shield of gold, from which golden rays are shining. Lift your hands away very slowly, little by little . . . see how the rays of light follow the movements of your hands. Using the power of your hands to direct the light, make a great golden shell that completely surrounds you. . . . It's as if you were inside an enormous egg made of golden light.

Explore the boundaries of this protective egg and you will find you can extend them as you please. Make the egg get bigger but also stronger. Understand that inside this shell you are completely safe, completely protected; the golden light is impenetrable and nothing can pass through it. Look, here comes a fly. . . . It's trying to bother you, it wants to land on you . . . but it can't get to you, it can't get through the golden egg.

Now I'm going to stop talking for a few moments and, all you will hear is the sweet sound of soft music. Nestle in your golden egg and feel how peaceful and comforting it is. Bathe in the light that surrounds you.

When you are ready to come back, open your eyes slowly and gently. Although you cannot see it with your eyes open, your golden shell is still around you, keeping you safe, protecting you: It is yours now and forever.

THE MAGIC ROOM
VISUALIZATION

Lie down and get comfortable. Don't cross your arms or legs. Relax completely, letting all the tension seep out of your muscles. Let it all go. Feel your body soften and loosen. Now close your eyes—gently, not tightly—and take three deep, slow breaths . . . one . . . two . . . three. . . .

Now that you are completely relaxed, get ready to go to a place that is all your own. This will be a place only you can go, because it is the creation of your mind.

To arrive at this place you must walk down a stairway of many colors. Step down onto the first, red stair: Something red is lying on it. I don't know what it is, but if you stoop down and look closely, you will see it clearly, you will know what it is. Now step down onto the second step, which is orange, and something orange is on it. See what it is. Step down onto the yellow stair, and notice the yellow object you find there. Now you are on the green step, looking at a green thing—only you know what it is. And now step down onto the blue step, with its object, entirely blue. Now you're on the indigo step, with something indigo on it—see what it is. Now you've come to the last, violet step. What violet thing do you find there?

Without opeing your eyes, look around at where you've ended up, and search for a suitable spot on which to construct your secret place. Your secret place could be a cabin or a castle, a bird's nest or a cloud, a tree or a giant flower—but don't do what I say, make something all your own. With the power of your thought you can create anything you want.

When you are sure you've found the right spot, use your hands—always keeping your eyes closed—to create your working space. This is a magic room, a magic space: Everything you want is right here, everything you might ever need. Do you want to watch cartoons? Snap your fingers and a television will instantly appear and play anything you want to see. Have you always wanted a cat or a dog? Snap your fingers and a cat or a dog will appear.

Now two people walk into your room, one male and one female. They are your helpers, they are here to give you a hand, and you can send them anywhere you wish by the power of your thought.

Look at the male being: Who is he? Is he a man or a boy or an animal or something else entirely? Greet him and thank him for coming to help you. Snap your fingers for a chair so that he can sit down.

Now look at the female being: Who or what is she? Do you know her or not? Is she little or big? Make another chair appear. Greet her and thank her for coming.

Make friends with your two helpers; you'll see that they will serve you well. Do you want to put them to work? They will always obey you. Ask them, for example, to bring you a magic globe that sends out colored lights. Watch how they disappear for a moment; watch how they come right back with the globe in their hands, lights of many colors spilling through their fingers.

Do you want to help someone? Do you want to give someone a special lift? Think of that person, and send your helpers out to bathe them in a ray of light into which you put your love. Choose the color of your ray of light. To send energy and strength, send a red, orange, or yellow ray. To soothe and send thoughts of peace, send a blue, indigo, or violet ray. A green ray is good for everything.

Your helpers travel at the speed of thought, so whenever you are worried or anxious about someone, you can send your helpers right to them with a ray of light full of love.

In your magic room there is a cupboard full of beautiful bottles of every color in the rainbow, and in these bottles are remedies for anything that ails you. Do you have a stomachache? Send one of your helpers to the cupboard to prepare you a potion. Did you hurt your knee? In one of the bottles is a special cream that will make it stop hurting. Are you scared of a school test? Your helpers will find the bottle that holds a liquid to make you brave.

There is a shower of light in your room that you can stand under when you are tired. Stand under it now and feel the light cascade down your body, filling it with energy and strength.

There is a bathtub filled with a softer light in your room as well, which you can climb into just to relax or when you want to fall asleep. Climb into it now and lie back. Feel how the light cradles you and supports you. Trust it completely. Let yourself feel the peacefulness of this light.

Anytime you are tired, you can come and stand under that shower. Anytime you need to relax, you can climb into that bathtub and lie back.

Anytime you want to, now and forever, you can come to this magic room, with its potions, its helpers, it rays, and showers and tubs of light. This is your place and it will always be here for you.

When you are ready, slowly open your eyes, stretch, and sit up. Notice how you feel full of energy, yet completely relaxed.

A Cautionary Postscript about the Magic Room

Magic has its own unbendable rules. And so you should know that your magic room and its helpers and potions and lights can only be used for good. So, no tripping up a kid you don't like; no tickling the teacher's nose and making it itch! Only positive things can be done with this magic, and anyone who cheats has to pay. It's the law of the boomerang: Everything comes back around. If you send out love, goodwill, and kind and helpful thoughts, the same will come to you. But if you send out disrespectful and spiteful thoughts . . . what do you think you'll get in return? Remember the rules of magic and always use your magic room wisely and well.

APPENDIX

CHILDREN'S RIGHTS

A charter of children's rights, like citizens' rights, already exists, but these rights are not always honored. It goes without saying that they have the right to be fed, housed, washed, cared for, and educated; but I think the first right of any child is to be happy. Love is our birthright, and although many misunderstand it, not one of us can live without it. Some of us, having been taught to do so as children, continue to limp along without much love in our lives for years, out of habit.

What does this have to do with Bach flowers? Dr. Bach acted on his convictions about all our rights to love, happiness, and health without violence. His sensitivity to this issue led him to abandon "violent" therapy in all forms—most heretically, the notorious "shot." He refused to use any substance that had to be injected. If children were writing their own Magna Carta, the right not to be stuck with sharp needles would surely be on it!

Dr. Bach pointed out more than once that every child must be free to follow whatever path nature indicates, whether it be repairing shoes or writing poems, pursuing physics or working in the garden. He insisted that we must not intervene with criticism or judgment when a child is expressing his or her creativity.

Yet how many times have we all stepped in to say things like, "Why did you draw the window so small?" or "The sun isn't pink!" or "Where are this little girl's arms?" Without meaning to, we discourage our budding artists. In the best-case scenario, they will modify their creation to content us; in the worst, they will destroy the drawing or be blocked in their artistic expression altogether. Children are always seeking to please us, to adapt so that they may continue to be acceptable in our eyes.

It can't hurt to say, "How beautiful! I can see you've worked very hard on this—what lovely colors you've used! I'll hang it up right away." With all due respect to modern art, we spend millions on abstract paintings; why not reward our children's artistic creations as well?

Another fundamental need and birthright of children is laughter. In our society we laugh ever less and depend more and more on the empty canned laughter of film or TV. The joy of finding life funny, of laughing all by ourselves, of creating reasons to laugh is a whole different thing. Laughter purifies the aura and strengthens the being. A sense of humor helps us to bear the heaviest burdens. It does us no damage, is not addictive, has no contraindications, and boosts our energies—just like Bach flowers!

Children also have the right to wear what they like rather than what pleases us, to choose their own colors and dress in clothes loose and comfortable enough to move around in, to play, climb, roll, and sit on the grass in without being shadowed by the fear of dirtying their "brand-new" or "special" clothes and angering their parents. Although we all succumb to the temptation sometimes, children are not dolls to dress up; they must have a voice in the matter. There are limits, of course: A bikini at New Year's won't do unless you're in Santo Domingo. But be generous with your aesthetics; the same combination of a red shirt and pink pants that gives you the willies may make them feel happy all day.

Ask your children whether they are warm or cold and try to evaluate the amount of clothing they should wear with realism. Parents often overdress their children, for some reason. I've seen parents in T-shirts hand-in-hand with sweaty little bundled-up snowmen. Remember that though they may have to walk to school in the morning or wait for the bus in the cold, schools themselves are often overheated. Dress them in layers they can remove as they warm up.

Children have the right to be believed. We needn't start from the presupposition that only adults tell the truth. Since their perspectives are so very different from ours, we would do well to analyze things from their point of view as well as our own. I have found that the more children are trusted, the more trustworthy they become.

Children have the right to rest, to take a break now and then. Have you ever had a day when you felt like you just couldn't go to work? I certainly have, and children experience this, too. Ignoring it, as we ourselves should know, can trigger a true illness for the reprieve it brings. How much better to declare a day of rest and respite, a special holiday of relaxation and renewal. Only you, knowing your children as well as you do, will know when to say: "I can see that you're very tired. Maybe tomorrow instead of going to school, you should sleep a little later than usual, and then we could take a walk in the park and enjoy the bright sunshine." A day lost from school won't set your child back and, as we know, the need to rest doesn't always coincide with the weekend.

I'd like to digress for a moment and, using this case as an example, illustrate the dynamics of the Bach flower system. An Oak child, in this situation, will refuse to relinquish her duty and insist on going to school, tired or not, while a Clematis child will agree right away, evasion being his creed. A Hornbeam child will show clear symptoms of physical and mental fatigue and will have a hard time waking up in the morning, while an Elm child will not feel up to the heavy burdens she feels she's carrying. Larch would just as soon run away from everything, anyway. Mimulus is afraid of being found out, and Pine feels guilty.

This is the lovely simplicity of Dr. Bach's method. You start with a situation and examine it from different angles, according to the child's way of being and reacting. Once you have familiarized yourselves with the system, all will go smoothly; all you have to do is make sure your evaluations are objective.

Our children have the very needs and rights that we have, which all too often we ignore. You will find that if you have fulfilled your needs for self-respect, affirmative thought, rest, laughter, hugs and kisses, love, tenderness, sharing, friendship, and collaboration, the children you care for, breathing deeply of your positivity, will also walk in health and balance of mind and body, at peace with themselves and the life around them.

This is a clear invitation, of course, to experiment on yourselves with the Bach flower remedies, which are such bearers of authentic balance and health. But be careful! You can get used to well-being, even addicted: Once you've felt really good for a while, it's hard to go back.

A Final Note
to Parents

I would like to spend a few moments dispelling any fears you might have about your capacity to administer these flower essences. Dr. Bach has reassured us that the principle and method are simple in the extreme. Much that springs from nature is so simple that we sometimes hesitate to place our faith in it, but it is we humans who are always complicating things.

Use these remedies fearlessly. You will see that once you familiarize yourselves with the flowers, carefully reading the descriptions and trusting your parental intuitions, you can hardly go wrong. And if you do make a mistake, as I've said before, no harm will come of it; none of these essences has damaging effects if wrongly administered. At the worst, nothing will happen, and you will have to try again and experiment.

If you feel too insecure to administer them to your children, take Larch and Cerato yourselves. If you are impatient to see results, take Impatiens.

If you expect gratitude in exchange for your efforts, take Chicory. What we do for our children we must do without thought of recompense; it is reward enough to have given life to these amazing beings who have come to teach us as well as to learn from us. We must not consider our children to be our private property or burden them by complaining about our efforts on their behalf. Unconditional love must be the very foundation of our relations with them—love for love's sake, without expectation. It is wrong to speak of the "sacrifices" we've made for them; the choice was ours.

Remember that all we do, whether positive or negative, comes back to us a thousandfold in many forms. Once we really understand this simple but ironclad law, we will have resolved many of our problems.

Inside each of us is the answer to every question; all we need to do is be silent and listen. This is how Dr. Bach found the flowers—by heeding his own intuitions and the world of nature, of which we are part. Once you begin using this system, you will see how simple it is to choose and administer a certain remedy. Trust your inner voice. I cannot emphasize enough that this method is intuitive, based more on sensitivity than on statistics. When it is backed by love, it cannot fail.

U.S. Supplier of
Bach Flower Remedies

The following company is the main distributor of Bach flower supplies in the United States and sells retail, as well as wholesale, by mail order.

Nelson Bach USA
100 Research Dr.
Wilmington, MA 01887
Phone: (978) 988-3833
Fax: (978) 988-0233

QUICK-REFERENCE TABLE OF REMEDIES

Disturbances/Issues	Causes/Conditions	Remedies
Abandonment	Fear of being abandoned	Red Chestnut
	Victim of actual abandonment	Star of Bethlehem
Aggression	Due to resentment, anger, or jealousy	Holly
	Due to desire for power	Vine
	Due to tension, temper, and explosive tantrums	Cherry Plum
	Critical and judgmental	Beech
Agitation	From anxiety and fear	Aspen or Mimulus
	Caused by enthusiasm	Vervain
	Due to hurry and impatience	Impatiens
	After trauma	Rescue Remedy or Star of Bethlehem
Anger	Manifest	Holly
	Veiled and repressed	Willow
Apology	Apologizes constantly	Pine
	Never apologizes	Holly
	Does not "have to" apologize for anything	Willow
	Thinks he/she is never in the wrong	Vine
	Expects apologies from others	Beech
	Shuts out others instead of apologizing	Water Violet
	Thinks him/herself incapable of making a mistake	Rock Water

Appetite	Lack of appetite and interest in food	Wild Rose or Clematis
	Refusal to eat as rebellion	Holly
	Problematic, due to desire to be the center of attention	Heather
	Manipulative, used as a means to obtain something	Chicory
	Voracious and exaggerated overeating	Vervain
	Secretive and addictive eating	Agrimony
	Frenetic and rushed overeating	Impatiens
	Overeating to fill emotional voids	Heather
	Overeating due to passive dissatisfaction	Wild Oat
Arrogance	Dominant and dictatorial	Vine
	Quarrelsome and hypercritical	Beech
	Fueled by anger	Holly
	Due to haste and disrespect for others	Impatiens
	Interfering due to nosiness	Chicory
	Due to desire to impose one's own ideas on others	Vervain
	Due to machismo	Vine
Asthma	In addition to bronchial, or while waiting for medical treatment	Rock Rose + Crab Apple + Centaury + Mimulus + Walnut or Gentian + Willow
	From allergens, as a preventive in addition to medical treatment	

Disturbances/Issues	Causes/Conditions	Remedies
Attachment to Bottle	Inability to relinquish bottle	Red Chestnut + Walnut + Honeysuckle
	Secretive attachment to bottle	Agrimony + Flowers above
Bedwetting	Due to daytime tension and witholding followed by nighttime "loosening"	Cherry Plum
	Due to severe anxiety masked by apparent serenity	Agrimony
	Due to regression or trauma	Star of Bethlehem
	Due to birth of a sibling	Holly
Blows and Shocks	Physical blows (apply topically to the bruise)	Rescue Cream
	Shock due to fear	Rescue Remedy
Blushing	Due to shyness or shame	Mimulus
Boredom	Accompanied by apathy	Wild Rose
	Inability to enjoy the present moment	Clematis
	Accompanied by repetitive action	Chestnut Bud
	Due to copying other people	Cerato
	Due to lack of real interests	Wild Oat
	Bores others by talking all the time	Heather
Colitis	As a symptom of fear	Aspen or Mimulus
	Due to uneasiness; excessively picky with food	Crab Apple

Death	Due to hurry and too fast a pace	Impatiens
	Fear of death	Aspen
	Terror of death	Rock Rose
	Death of a loved one	Gentian, Gorse
	Despair following death of a loved one	Sweet Chestnut
	To be administered to the dying	Honeysuckle + Gorse
	To be administered to those assisting the dying	Rescue Remedy
Diffidence	Accompanied by hostility	Holly
	Accompanied by criticism	Beech
	Accompanied by pessimism	Willow
	For fear of the new and unknown	Mimulus
	Because of distrust	Larch
Distraction	Head in the clouds	Clematis
	Learning-impaired	Chestnut Bud
	Mentally tired	Hornbeam
	Lacking in interest	Wild Oat + Wild Rose
Drowsiness	Due to spaciness, lack of being present in the moment	Clematis
	Due to apathy and lack of will	Wild Rose
	In the morning, with difficulty waking up	Hornbeam
	Due to being overtired or weakened by illness	Olive
	Due to passivity and dissatisfaction	Wild Oat

Disturbances/Issues	Causes/Conditions	Remedies
Ears	Disturbances in equilibrium	Scleranthus
	Disturbances due to loud noise	Mimulus
	Disturbances due to hypersensitivity	Clematis
	Problems with hearing	Clematis
	Problems with hearing and balance	Scleranthus
Egotism	Demanding, center of the universe	Heather
	Wants a lot in exchange for right action	Chicory
	Self-pitying,	
	feels a reward is due him or her, gives very little	Willow
	Enjoys power-tripping	Vine
	Feels victimized by others	Centaury
Emergencies	While waiting for medical treatment	Rescue Remedy or Rock Rose
Envy	Inner feelings of envy	Holly
	Envy manifested as copying others	Cerato
Exhaustion	Physical, from overwork	Oak
	Mental, in need of rest and renewal	Hornbeam
	Physical and mental,	
	or when convalescing from illness	Olive
	Nervous, due to burdens carried in the psyche	Cherry Plum

	After a trauma or disappointment	Rescue Remedy + Gentian + Olive
	With inexplicable depression	Mustard
	Accompanied by apathy and resignation	Wild Rose
Failure	Trauma from recent failure	Gentian or Gorse
	A constant sense of oneself as a failure	Larch
	Lack of recovery from past failure	Star of Bethlehem
	Sense of failure due to too much responsibility	Elm
Fear	Of known cause	Mimulus
	Vague and intangible, cause unknown	Aspen
	Anxious in nature	Aspen
	Terror and panic	Rock Rose
	For the safety of others	Red Chestnut
	Repressed, maniacal, held tightly under control	Cherry Plum
	Anguished and hidden from others	Agrimony
	Of night	Rock Rose + Aspen
Fever	While waiting for medical attention	Rescue Remedy + Hornbeam
	In sickness, with itching and rash	Crab Apple and Rescue Cream
	Accompanied by prostration	Rescue Remedy + Olive
	Accompanied by pain in the joints	Rescue Remedy + (according to type) Beech, Vine, Water Violet, Rock Water, Pine, Vervain, Holly

Disturbances/Issues	Causes/Conditions	Remedies
Fright	At the moment of fright	Rescue Remedy or Rock Rose
	After a fright	Star of Bethlehem
	To help confront something frightening	Rescue Remedy + Larch + Gentian
Gifts	To which too much importance is given	Chicory
	Obtained by conscious manipulation	Chicory
	That must equal those received by others	Cerato
	That must always be the same	Chestnut Bud
	That mean so much	
	he/she does not dare ask for them	Centaury
	So that they may be given freely to others	Agrimony
	That are demanded	Heather
Gluttony	Due to lack of affection	Heather or Chicory
	Due to anger	Holly
	Due to inner anguish leading to addiction	Agrimony
	Due to dissatisfaction	Wild Oat
	Due to erroneous habits	Walnut
Handicaps	To overcome discouragement	Gorse
	due to chronic handicap or illness	
	To acquire and strengthen faith	Larch + Cerato

To help in learning and recovery	Chestnut Bud
To ease the burdens of psychosis	Elm + Cherry Plum
In nervous crises and breakdowns	Cherry Plum
For trembling due to anxiety	Aspen
In cases of Down's syndrome	Chestnut Bud
In cases of autism	Chestnut Bud + Rock Water + Sweet Chestnut
To reawaken interest	Wild Rose, Wild Oat, or Clematis
In cases of obsession	Cherry Plum or Crab Apple
In cases of hypersensitivity	Walnut, Mimulus, or Centaury
In cases of hyperkinesis	Impatiens
To reduce spasticity	Rock Water, Pine, White Chestnut, or Beech
Hatred	
Accompanied by anger, envy, and jealousy	Holly
Accompanied by rancor and hostility	Willow
Of oneself	Pine
Of oneself, along with a sense of shame and "dirtiness"	Crab Apple
Headaches and Migraines	
Due to intense mental activity and brooding	White Chestnut
Due to uneasiness and feelings of inferiority	Pine
Due to excessive TV or music, resulting in "heavy head" and sometimes fever	Hornbeam

Disturbances/Issues	Causes/Conditions	Remedies
Hyperactivity	Hurries through everything	Impatiens
	With tension and mental agitation, sometimes accompanied by maniacal gestures	Cherry Plum
	With mental agitation caused by obsessive thinking	White Chestnut
	With overinvolvement, exaggeration, and abuse of energy	Vervain
	Overworking without complaint	Oak
	Due to too much to do	Elm
	Due to anger coupled with destruction and rebellion	Holly
Hysteria	Due to tension, with sudden outbursts of rage	Cherry Plum
	To attract attention	Chicory
	Due to anger	Holly
	Due to fear and panic	Rock Rose, Star of Bethlehem, or (better yet) Rescue Remedy
Illness	As a means to attract attention	Heather, Willow, or Chicory
	Cyclic illnesses	Chestnut Bud
	Slow recovery rate	Clematis + Wild Rose
	To restore optimism	Agrimony

	Fear of illness	Aspen, Mimulus, or Crab Apple
	Rashes	Rescue Remedy + Crab Apple + Agrimony
	Illnesses with catarrh	Crab Apple
	Debilitating illness	Olive
	Chronic illness	Gorse
	Illness from which recovery seems impossible	Star of Bethlehem
Imbalance	Physical, accompanied by dizzyness	Scleranthus
	Emotional mood swings	Scleranthus
	Loss of balance, even falling due to distraction	Clematis
	Bumping into things due to frenetic pace	Impatiens
Impatience	As a basic personality trait	Impatiens
	Inability to conclude projects	Chestnut Bud
Impulsivity	General	Impatiens or Vervain
Indecision	Due to psychological and physical exhaustion	Olive
	Due to meager interest	Wild Rose
Insomnia	For fear of ghosts and darkness	Aspen
	Due to inability to quiet the mind	White Chestnut
	Due to hyperactivity and frenetic biorhythms	Impatiens or Vervain
	Due to melancholy	Mustard

171

Disturbances/Issues	Causes/Conditions	Remedies
Insomnia (*cont.*)	Due to homesickness	Honeysuckle
	Due to secret anguish	Agrimony
	Due to intense nervous tension	Cherry Plum
	For fear of being guilty	Pine
	To get attention	Heather
	Due to resentment	Willow
Jealousy	Expressed or unexpressed	Holly
	Accompanied by possessiveness	Chicory
Mental Confusion	Due to excessive activity and hurry	Impatiens
	Due to distraction	Clematis
	Due to distraction that impairs learning	Clematis + Chestnut Bud
	Due to overenthusiasm and exaggeration	Vervain
	Due to indecision	Scleranthus
	Due to passivity;	
	initiates but never brings to completion	Wild Oat
	Due to lack of faith in the self	Cerato
Menstruation	Fear of menarche	Mimulus
	Experienced as dirty or impure	Crab Apple

Monsters	Accompanied by pain	Star of Bethlehem
	Accompanied by terror	Rock Rose
	Kept secret, for fear	Aspen
	Fear of the dead	Rock Rose + Aspen
	Fascination with/fear of monsters	Aspen
	Experienced as real	Mimulus
Morning	Has a hard time waking up	Hornbeam
	Wakes up very early in a state of anxiety	Aspen
	Fusses about going to school	Honeysuckle
Nausea	In general	Scleranthus
	Due to indigestion	Crab Apple
Nightmares	General	Rock Rose
	Accompanied by sleepwalking	Rock Rose + Aspen
Odors	Smells are experienced as irritating	Mimulus
	Smells are experienced as repulsive and "dirty"	Crab Apple
Pain	Due to growing	Elm
	Due to unknown causes	Pine
	Due to rigidity	Beech, Rock Water, or Water Violet
	Due to stress	Vervain, Impatiens, Oak, or Elm
	Feigned	Willow, Chicory, or Heather

Disturbances/Issues	Causes/Conditions	Remedies
Parent(s)	Inability to let go of mother/father	Walnut + Red Chestnut
	Homesickness for mother/father	Honeysuckle
	Inability to do anything without mother/father	Larch + Cerato
	Fear that mother/father will die	Aspen + Red Chestnut
	Suffocating mother/father	Centaury
	Fear of saying "no" to mother/father	Centaury
Passivity	Due to drowsiness and excessive quiet	Clematis
	Due to lifelessness and lack of interest	Wild Rose
	Due to follower mentality and	Centaury
	submissiveness	
	Due to resignation	Gorse
Perfectionism	Manifested as inflexibility with oneself	Rock Water
	Meticulous and pedantic	Crab Apple
	Accompanied by the expectation of	
	perfection in others	Beech
	Manifested as fussy, busybody behavior	Chicory
Pessimism	Due to lack of faith in the self	Cerato
	Due to a sense of failure	Larch
	Due to discouragement and doubt	Gentian
	Accompanied by veiled rancor	Willow

Pimples	Due to need for systemic cleansing	Crab Apple
	Experienced as "dirty"	Crab Apple
	Due to repressed rage	Holly
	Due to emotional eruption	Impatiens
Possessiveness	Manipulative	Chicory
	Accompanied by desire	Holly
	Coupled with domination	Vine
School	First day of	Honeysuckle + Walnut
	Fear of	Mimulus
	Exhaustion from overwork	Elm
	Distrust of	Larch
	Distraction during	Clematis
	Difficulty learning; repetition of errors	Chestnut Bud
	Requires constant confirmation	Cerato
	Does not feel respected or appreciated	Centaury
	Attends class even when sick	Oak
Snacks	Devoured in secret	Agrimony + Walnut
	Snacking due to lack of interest in other food	Wild Rose
	Snacking to fill a void and deal with boredom	Wild Oat
Speech	Feeble, as if it were blocked	Star of Bethlehem
	Low and sweet but barely audible	Water Violet
	Oratorical, loud, high, and decisive	Vervain

Disturbances/Issues	Causes/Conditions	Remedies
Speech (cont.)	Strident and hysterical	Holly or Cherry Plum
	Blocked by inner anxiety	Aspen
	Low murmuring due to shyness	Mimulus
	Paralyzed, unable to speak	Rock Rose
	Harsh and peremptory, bossy	Vine
	Continuous, nonsensical speech	Heather
	Difficulty speaking due to anxiety	Aspen
	Difficulty speaking due to nervous tension	Cherry Plum
	Difficulty speaking due to immaturity	Chestnut Bud
	Difficulty speaking due to rush and impatience	Impatiens
Stammering	Due to shyness	Mimulus
	Due to inner tension	Cherry Plum
	Due to lack of self-confidence	Larch
Tantrums	Shouting, in a violent crisis of rage	Cherry Plum
	Breaking things and stamping feet	Holly
	Whining to get one's way	Chicory
	Despotic, for personal power	Vine
Teething	During teething	Walnut
	Painful and anguished teething	Walnut + Agrimony
	Painful teething with exhaustion	Walnut + Agrimony + Olive

Tension	Held under tight control; sometimes explosive	Cherry Plum
	Due to haste and fast-paced rhythm	Impatiens
	Due to energy wasted trying to convince others of one's own convictions	Vervain
	Due to emotional repression and isolation from others	Water Violet
	Due to the need to be boss	Vine
	Inner, hidden from others	Agrimony
	Due to worrying about others	Red Chestnut
	Due to anxiety about the future	Aspen
	Due to need to set an example	Rock Water
	Due to need to be heard	Heather
Throat	Lump in the throat	Aspen, Water Violet, Star of Bethlehem, Centaury, Mustard, Mimulus, or Rock Rose
Tongue, Coated	Due to indigestion	Crab Apple + Elm + Chicory
	Due to poor diet	Crab Apple + Walnut + Agrimony
Torment	Due to nervous disturbance	Cherry Plum
	Inner, hidden by apparent gaiety	Agrimony
	Due to jealousy	Chicory
	Torments others	Vine
	Due to self-punishment and blame	Pine

Disturbances/Issues	Causes/Conditions	Remedies
Transitions	For difficulties accompanying all states of transition	Walnut
	When accompanied by nostalgia	Walnut + Honeysuckle
Weeping	Hysterical and uncontrollable	Cherry Plum
	Angry and irritable	Holly
	Accompanied by whining	Chicory
	During temper tantrums	Chicory
	Weak and submissive	Star of Bethlehem
	Resigned	Wild Rose
	From exhaustion	Olive
	To be the center of attention	Heather
	Because of disappointed expectations	Vervain
	Secretive and silent	Water Violet
	Because of being blamed or feeling guilty	Pine
	Due to minimized or unexpressed inner anguish	Agrimony
Whininess	"Nothing ever goes right"	Gentian + Willow
	Critical of others	Beech
	Fixates on things	Rock Water
	Annoying and repetitive	Chestnut Bud

INDEX